The 2x2 Matrix

A. J. Larner

The 2x2 Matrix

Contingency, Confusion and the Metrics
of Binary Classification

Second Edition

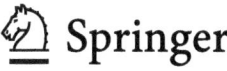 Springer

A. J. Larner
Cognitive Function Clinic
Walton Centre for Neurology
and Neurosurgery
Liverpool, UK

Department of Brain Repair
and Rehabilitation
Institute of Neurology
University College London
London, UK

ISBN 978-3-031-47193-3   ISBN 978-3-031-47194-0 (eBook)
https://doi.org/10.1007/978-3-031-47194-0

1st edition: © Springer Nature Switzerland AG 2021
2nd edition: © The Editor(s) (if applicable) and The Author(s), under exclusive license to Springer
Nature Switzerland AG 2024

This Springer imprint is published by the registered company Springer Nature Switzerland AG
The registered company address is: Gewerbestrasse 11, 6330 Cham, Switzerland

Paper in this product is recyclable.

Preface to the Second Edition

The principles underpinning this second edition remain the same as in the first: to describe, extend, and illustrate (through worked examples) the many available measures used in binary classification. (In this context, the title of "metrics" uses the word in its common usage, as synonymous with "measures," and not in its mathematical definition of satisfying the triangle inequality, in the light of which not all the measures discussed here are metrics, e.g. F measure; Sect. 4.8.3. [1]). As previously, the basis for most of the worked examples is the dataset of a screening test accuracy study of the Mini-Addenbrooke's Cognitive Examination (MACE) administered in a dedicated clinic for the diagnosis of cognitive disorders.

The whole text has been revised, involving some reorganisation of material. Specific new material includes:

- A section devoted to the interrelations of Sens, Spec, PPV, NPV, P, and Q (Chap. 2), as well as the expression of other measures in terms of P and Q, such as Y, PSI, HMYPSI, MCC, CSI, and F (Chap. 4).
- Introduction of the recently described Efficiency index and its extensions (Chap. 5).
- Sections on balanced and unbiased measures have been added, for accuracy (Chap. 3), identification index (Chap. 4), and Efficiency index (Chap. 5).
- Discussion of the (thorny) issue of "diagnostic yield" (Chap. 4).
- More on the number needed (reciprocal) measures and their combination as likelihoods, including new metrics: number needed to classify correctly, number needed to misclassify, likelihood to classify correctly or misclassify (Chap. 5).
- The previously scattered material on "quality" metrics has been brought together and treated systematically in a new chapter (Chap. 6).
- More on the classification of the various metrics of binary classification (meta-classification) and on fourfold classifications more generally (Chap. 9).

The audience for the book, as before, is potentially very broad and may include any researcher or clinician or professional allied to medicine who uses or plans to use measures of binary classification, for example for diagnostic or screening instruments. In addition, the metrics described may be pertinent to fields such as informatics, data searching and machine learning, and any discipline involving predictions (e.g. ecology, meteorology, analysis of administrative datasets).

The Scottish Enlightenment philosopher David Hume (1711–1776) in his *Philosophical Essays* of 1748 (First Enquiry, Part 4, Sect. 1) wrote that:

> All the Objects of human Reason or Enquiry may naturally be divided into two kinds, *viz. Relations of Ideas*, and *Matters of Fact*. Of the first Kind are the Propositions in Geometry, Algebra, and Arithmetic … [which are] discoverable by the mere operation of thought … Matters of Fact, which are the second Objects of human Reason, are not ascertain'd to us in the same Manner; nor is our Evidence of their Truth, however great, of a like Nature with the foregoing. The contrary of every Matter of Fact is still possible; … (cited in [2], p.253, 427n.xii).

The material presented here, being largely arithmetical and, to a lesser extent, graphical, may be considered to fall into Hume's category of *Relations of Ideas* and hence definitionally or necessarily true because purely logical. However, by using empirical datasets to illustrate these operations, the outcomes may also be considered as at least putative *Matters of Fact* (if the calculations have been performed correctly!) and hence contingent because dependent on evidence. Thus, whilst the latter may be contradicted or rejected in the light of further evidence, the former, the *Relations of Ideas*, will persist and, dependent upon their perceived utility, be applicable in any situation where binary classification is used.

Liverpool, UK   A. J. Larner

Acknowledgements My thanks are due to Elizabeth Larner who drew Figs. 8.6 and 9.1–9.4. Also to Dr. Gashirai Mbizvo with whom I have collaborated productively in work on CSI and F (Chap. 4) and the ROC plot (Chap. 7). All errors or misconceptions expressed in this work are solely my own.

References

1. Powers DMW. What the F measure doesn't measure … Features, flaws, fallacies and fixes. 2015. https://arxiv.org/abs/1503.06410.2015.
2. Wootton D. The invention of science. A new history of the scientific revolution. London: Penguin; 2016.

Preface to the First Edition

It is important to state at the outset what this book is not. It is not a textbook of medical statistics, as I have no training, far less any expertise, in that discipline. Rather it is a heuristic, based on experience of using and developing certain mathematical operations in the context of evaluating the outcomes of diagnostic and screening test accuracy studies. It therefore stands at the intersection of different disciplines, borrowing from them (a dialogic discourse?) in the hope that the resulting fusion or intermingling will result in useful outcomes. This reflects part of a wider commitment to interdisciplinary studies [6, 16].

Drawing as they do on concepts derived from decision theory, signal detection theory, and Bayesian methods, 2×2 contingency tables may find application in many areas, for example medical decision-making, weather forecasting, information retrieval, machine learning and data mining. Of necessity, this volume is written from the perspective of the first of these areas, as the author is a practising clinician, but nevertheless it contains much material which will be of relevance to a wider audience.

Accordingly, this book is a distillate of what I have found to be helpful as a clinician working in the field of test accuracy studies, specifically related to the screening and diagnosis of dementia and cognitive impairment, undertaken in the context of a dedicated cognitive disorders clinic. The conceptual framework described here is supplemented with worked examples in each section of the book, over 60 in all, since, to quote Edwin Abbott, "An instance will do more than a volume of generalities to make my meaning clear" ([1], p. 56). Many of these examples are based on a large (N = 755) pragmatic prospective screening test accuracy study of one particular brief cognitive screening instrument, the Mini-Addenbrooke's Cognitive Examination (MACE) [3], the use of which in my clinical work has been extensively analysed and widely presented [7–9, 11–15]. (It has also been included in a systematic review of MACE [2]). Further analyses of MACE are presented here, along with material from some of the other studies which have been undertaken in the clinic [4]. My previous books documenting the specifics of such pragmatic test accuracy studies of cognitive screening instruments [5, 10] may be categorised as parerga, the current work being more general in scope and hence applicable to many branches of medical decision-making as well as to disciplines beyond medicine wherein the binary classification is required. Statistical programmes are not discussed.

James Clerk Maxwell (1831–1879) believed that there was "a department of the mind conducted independently of consciousness" where ideas could be "fermented and decocted so that when they run off they come clear" ([17], p. 94–5, 154), views with which I am largely in agreement (clarity of my own ideas, however, seldom being apparent). This prompts me to acknowledge two periods of annual leave, both spent at Center Parcs, Whinfell Forest, Cumbria, which lead to the embryonic overall plan for this book (January 2019) and to the formulation of ideas about the epistemological matrix (November 2016).

Liverpool, UK   A. J. Larner

Acknowledgements Thanks are due to Alison Zhu, a proper mathematician (1st in mathematics from Trinity College Cambridge) for advising on many of the equations in this book, although I hasten to add that any remaining errors are solely my own. Thanks also to Elizabeth Larner who drew Fig. 7.7 [1st edition; Fig. 8.6 in 2nd edition].

References

1. Abbott EA. Flatland. An edition with notes and commentary by William F Lindgren and Thomas F Banchoff. New York: Cambridge University Press/Mathematical Association of America; [1884] 2010.
2. Beishon LC, Batterham AP, Quinn TJ, et al. Addenbrooke's Cognitive Examination III (ACEIII) and mini-ACE for the detection of dementia and mild cognitive impairment. Cochrane Database Syst Rev. 2019;12:CD013282. [There are several numerical errors relating to my data in this publication, viz.: P7, Summary of findings: PPV for MCI vs. none incorrect for both 21 and 25 test threshold; P17, Figure 8: Incorrect N (= 754!), TP, FP, TN. Figure 9: Incorrect TP, FP, FN; P18, Figure 10: Incorrect N (= 756!), FP. Figure 11: Incorrect TP, FP, TN; P29, Characteristics of individual studies: "22 with MCI" should read "222 with MCI"; P52, Appendix 6, Summary of included studies: "DSM-V" should read "DSM-IV".]
3. Hsieh S, McGrory S, Leslie F, Dawson K, Ahmed S, Butler CR, et al. The Mini-Addenbrooke's Cognitive Examination: a new assessment tool for dementia. Dement Geriatr Cogn Disord. 2015;39:1–11.
4. Larner AJ. Dementia in clinical practice: a neurological perspective. Pragmatic studies in the Cognitive Function Clinic. 3rd edition. London: Springer; 2018.
5. Larner AJ. Diagnostic test accuracy studies in dementia: a pragmatic approach. 2nd edition. London: Springer; 2019.
6. Larner AJ. Neuroliterature. Patients, doctors, diseases. Literary perspectives on disorders of the nervous system. Gloucester: Choir Press; 2019.
7. Larner A. MACE: optimal cut-offs for dementia and MCI. J Neurol Neurosurg Psychiatry. 2019;90:A19.
8. Larner AJ. MACE for diagnosis of dementia and MCI: examining cut-offs and predictive values. Diagnostics (Basel). 2019;9:E51.
9. Larner AJ. Applying Kraemer's Q (positive sign rate): some implications for diagnostic test accuracy study results. Dement Geriatr Cogn Dis Extra. 2019;9:389–96.

10. Larner AJ. Manual of screeners for dementia. Pragmatic test accuracy studies. London: Springer; 2020.
11. Larner AJ. Screening for dementia: Q* index as a global measure of test accuracy revisited. medRxiv. 2020; https://doi.org/10.1101/2020.04.01.20050567.
12. Larner AJ. Defining "optimal" test cut-off using global test metrics: evidence from a cognitive screening instrument. Neurodegener Dis Manag. 2020;10:223–30.
13. Larner AJ. Mini-Addenbrooke's Cognitive Examination (MACE): a useful cognitive screening instrument in older people? Can Geriatr J. 2020;23:199–204.
14. Larner AJ. Assessing cognitive screening instruments with the critical success index. Prog Neurol Psychiatry. 2021;25(3):33–7.
15. Larner AJ. Cognitive testing in the COVID-19 era: can existing screeners be adapted for telephone use? Neurodegener Dis Manag. 2021;11:77–82.
16. Larner AJ. Neuroliterature 2. Biography, semiology, miscellany. Further literary perspectives on disorders of the nervous system. In preparation.
17. Mahon B. The man who changed everything. The life of James Clerk Maxwell. Chichester:Wiley; 2004.

Contents

Chapter 1
Introduction

Contents

1.1 History and Nomenclature

Use of a fourfold or quadripartite 2 × 2 table to represent counts of different classes, a dichotomous classification, may date back to Aristotle [27]. Examples of the application of such tables to medical issues may be found in the work of Gavarret in the 1840s and Liebermeister in the 1870s [21, 27].

The term "contingency table" to describe a matrix format used to display a frequency distribution of variables is generally credited to Karl Pearson (1857–1936) in his lecture to the Draper's Society in 1904 [24]. Furthermore, in his book, *The grammar of science*, Pearson stated:

> ... all we can do is to classify things into like within a certain degree of observation, and record whether what we note as following from them are like within another degree of observation. Whenever we do this ... we really form a contingency table, ... (cited from the 3rd edition of *The grammar of science* [21], p.90-1).

Nevertheless, "contingency table" barely features in Porter's biography of Pearson ([25] p.266, 273).

The term "confusion matrix" or error matrix, or table of confusion, has also been applied to 2×2 tables, with the columns denoting instances of an actual class and the rows denoting instances of a predicted class. The term "confusion matrix" derives from the observation that this form of cross tabulation (or crosstab) makes it easy to see if the system is confusing two classes. The confusion matrix may be described as a special kind (2×2) of contingency table, since higher order contingency tables may be constructed, cross tabulating instances into more classes, represented by more columns and/or rows (see Sect. 8.5.1). Another term sometimes used to describe the 2×2 table is a "truth table", by analogy with those tables developed by the philosopher Ludwig Wittgenstein (1889–1951) for use in logic (see Sects. 1.3.1 and 8.2.2; Fig. 8.1).

The 2×2 contingency table or confusion matrix effectively entabulates chance and contingency, hence it reifies a binary system of classification. This should not, however, be confused with the binary or dyadic notation, using the base 2, the development of which is often associated (perhaps unjustifiably) with Gottfried Leibniz (1646–1716) [3].

The 2×2 contingency table is applicable to decision making in many disciplines. The details of this table are now described.

1.2   The Fourfold (2×2) Contingency Table

The simple 2×2 contingency table or confusion matrix cross-tabulates all instances (N) into classes, according to some form of reference standard or "true status" (e.g. diagnosis, or meteorological observations) in the vertical columns, against the outcome of a test or classifier of interest (e.g. a diagnostic or screening test, or meteorological forecasts) in the horizontal rows. In other words, there is a mapping of all instances to predicted classes, giving an indication of the performance of the classifier. The columns may be characterised as explanatory variables, the rows as response variables. This quadripartite classification thus categorises all individuals, observations, or events as:

- true positive (TP), or a "hit"
- false positive (FP), or a "false alarm" or "false hit"
- false negative (FN), or a "miss"
- true negative (TN), or a "non event" or "correct rejection"

These are the four outcomes recognised by the standard theory of signal detection [23]. Using the nomenclature of sets, these categories are disjoint sets.

This cross-classification is shown in a 2×2 contingency table in Fig. 1.1. Henceforward the terms TP, FP, FN, TN will be referred to as "literal notation", and measures derived from the 2×2 contingency table and denoted by equations using this notation will be referred to as "literal equations". Some readers may find such literal terminology easier to use and comprehend than algebraic notation.

The 2 × 2 table is often set out using algebraic terms, where:

- TP = a
- FP = b
- FN = c
- TN = d

This is shown in Fig. 1.2. Henceforward the terms a, b, c, d will be referred to as "algebraic notation", and equations using this notation as "algebraic equations". Some readers may find this algebraic terminology easier to use and comprehend than literal notation.

N is used throughout this book to denote the total number of instances observed or counted (e.g. patients or observations), in other words a population, such that:

		True Status	
		Condition present	**Condition absent**
Test Outcome	**Positive**	True positive [TP]	False positive [FP]
	Negative	False negative [FN]	True negative [TN]

Fig. 1.1.   2 × 2 contingency table using literal notation

		True Status	
		Condition present	**Condition absent**
Test Outcome	**Positive**	True positive (a)	False positive (b)
	Negative	False negative (c)	True negative (d)

Fig. 1.2.   2 × 2 contingency table using algebraic notation

$$N = TP + FP + FN + TN$$
$$= a + b + c + d$$

It should be noted, however, that some authors have used N to denote total negatives or negative instances (FN + TN, or c + d), for which the term q' is used here (see Sect. 1.3.1).

1.3   Marginal Totals and Marginal Probabilities

In any fourfold or quadripartite classification, the four terms can be paired in six possible combinations or permutations, expressed as either totals or probabilities, and these are exhaustive if combinations of two of the same kind are not permitted (if permitted, ten permutations would be possible).

1.3.1   Marginal Totals

It is immediately obvious that the four cells of the 2 × 2 table will generate six marginal values or totals by simple addition in the vertical, horizontal, and diagonal directions (Fig. 1.3). These totals will be denoted here using lower case letters.

Reading vertically, down the columns:

$$p = TP + FN = a + c$$
$$p' = FP + TN = b + d$$
$$p + p' = N$$

In other words, p = positive instances and p' = negative instances. This may also be illustrated in a simple truth table akin to that used in logic when using "p" and "–p" or "not p" for propositions (Fig. 1.4).

A dataset is said to be balanced when p = p'. A difference in these columnar marginal totals (i.e. in the numbers of positive, p, and negative, p', instances) is termed class imbalance. This may impact on the utility of some measures derived from the 2 × 2 contingency table.

Reading horizontally, across the rows:

$$q = TP + FP = a + b$$
$$q' = FN + TN = c + d$$
$$q + q' = N$$

In other words, q = positive classifications and q' = negative classifications.

		True Status		
		Condition present (= case)	Condition absent (= non case)	r'
Test Outcome	Positive	True positive [TP] (a)	False positive [FP] (b)	q
	Negative	False negative [FN] (c)	True negative [TN] (d)	q'
		p	p'	r

Marginal totals:

p	=	TP + FN	=	a + c
p'	=	FP + TN	=	b + d
p + p'	=	N	=	a + b + c + d
q	=	TP + FP	=	a + b
q'	=	FN + TN	=	c + d
q + q'	=	N	=	a + b + c + d
r	=	TP + TN	=	a + d
r'	=	FP + FN	=	b + c
r + r'	=	N	=	a + b + c + d

Marginal probabilities:

P	=	(TP + FN)/N	=	p/N
(1 − P) = P'	=	(FP + TN)/N	=	p'/N
Q	=	(TP + FP)/N	=	q/N
(1 − Q) = Q'	=	(FN + TN)/N	=	q'/N
R	=	(TP + TN)/N	=	r/N
(1 − R) = R'	=	(FP + FN)/N	=	r'/N

Fig. 1.3. 2×2 contingency table with marginal totals and marginal probabilities

It is also possible to read the table diagonally:

$$r = TP + TN = a + d$$
$$r' = FP + FN = b + c$$
$$r + r' = N$$

In other words, r = true instances and r' = false instances. (It should be noted that the use of "r" here has a different meaning from that used by other authors with respect to ratios of relevant costs, and in kappa values.) The sum of (TP + TN) has also been called "efficiency" ([11], p.27, 34, 115), and hence the sum of (FP + FN) may be termed "inefficiency" (see Sect. 5.11).

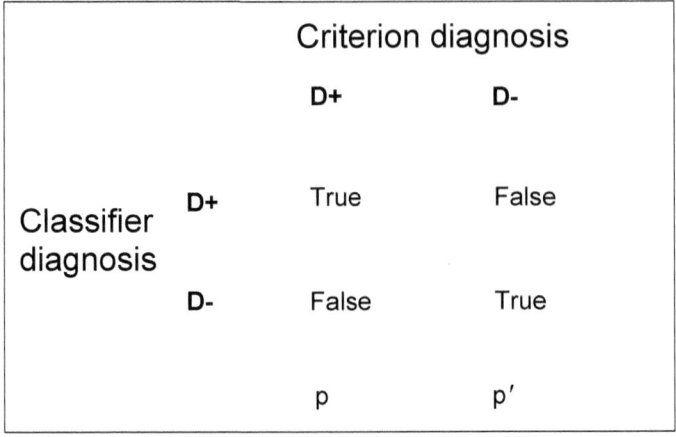

Fig. 1.4. 2 × 2 truth table for "p" and "not p" (or "–p")

Henceforward the terms p, p′, q, q′, r, and r′ will be referred to as marginal totals and will be substituted in some algebraic equations.

1.3.2 Marginal Probabilities; P, Q

The six absolute marginal totals may be converted to six probabilities, or rates, by dividing each by N. These probabilities or rates will be denoted using upper case letters.

Reading vertically in Fig. 1.3, there are two columnar ratios:

$$P = (TP + FN)/N = (a + c)/N = p/N$$
$$P' = (1 - P) = (FP + TN)/N = (b + d)/N = p'/N$$

As probabilities, these values necessarily sum to unity:

$$P + P' = 1$$

Using the nomenclature of sets, P′ is the complement of P, and P and P′ are disjoint sets. (Further examples of complementary parameters derived from the 2 × 2 contingency table will be encountered, in Chaps. 2 and 3.)

P is the prevalence, or prevalence rate, or base rate. When P = 0.5 there is a balanced class distribution (i.e. no class imbalance) because by definition P = P′ = 0.5.

P is used throughout this book to denote prevalence. It should be noted, however, that some authors use P to denote total positives or positive instances (TP + FP, or a + b), for which the term q is used here (Sect. 1.3.1).

Prevalence may also be expressed in probability notation, as the probability that disease is either present, the pre-test probability, $p(D+)$, or absent, $p(D-)$.

Worked Examples: Prevalence Rates (P, P′)

The Mini-Addenbrooke's Cognitive Examination (MACE) [10], a brief cognitive screening instrument, was subjected to a screening test accuracy study in a large patient cohort, N = 755 [13]. A reference (criterion) diagnosis of dementia, based on the application of widely accepted diagnostic criteria for dementia, was made in 114 patients. At the MACE cut-off of ≤20/30, the test outcomes were as follows: TP = 104, FN = 10, FP = 188, and TN = 453.

Hence the prevalence (P) or pre-test probability of dementia patients in this cohort was:

$$
\begin{aligned}
P &= (TP + FN)/N \\
&= (104 + 10)/755 \\
&= 0.151 \\
&= p(D+)
\end{aligned}
$$

The prevalence (P′) of patients without dementia, or pre-test probability against dementia, in the cohort was:

$$
\begin{aligned}
P' &= (FP + TN)/N \\
&= (188 + 453)/755 \\
&= 0.849 \\
&= 1 - P \\
&= p(D-)
\end{aligned}
$$

Prevalence may be a useful estimate of pre-test probability (see also Sect. 4.7) from which pre-test odds may be calculated (Sect. 1.3.3). However, sample prevalence may differ from population prevalence, and hence this base rate may be no more than an anchor from which to make adjustments (Sect. 3.4). Many of the measures derived from the 2 × 2 contingency table may be dependent on prevalence. This variation may be examined empirically, for example by using patient cohorts with different base rates of disease prevalence (e.g. [16, 17, 29], and [18], p.160, 165) or by calculation at fixed values of prevalence (Sects. 2.3.3 and 2.3.4) (e.g. [13, 18]).

Reading horizontally in Fig. 1.3, there are two row ratios:

$$
Q = (TP + FP)/N = (a + b)/N = q/N
$$

Hence Q may be described as the positive sign rate [11] or the probability of a positive test in the study population, or bias.

$$Q' = (1 - Q) = (FN + TN)/N = (c + d)/N = q'/N$$

Hence Q' may be described as the negative sign rate [14] or the probability of a negative test in the study population.

$$Q + Q' = 1$$

Using the nomenclature of sets, Q' is the complement of Q, and Q and Q' are disjoint sets. When $Q = 0$, all the negatives are correct but none of the positives ($Q' = 1$); when $Q = 1$, all of the positives are correct but none of the negatives ($Q' = 0$).

Q may also be expressed in probability notation, as the probability that the test is either positive, $p(T+)$, or negative, $p(T-)$.

Worked Examples: Positive and Negative Sign Rates (Q, Q′)

In the screening test accuracy study of (MACE) [13], from the patient cohort ($N = 755$) at the MACE cut-off of $\leq 20/30$, the test outcomes were as follows: TP = 104, FN = 10, FP = 188, and TN = 453.

Hence the positive sign rate (Q) at MACE cut-off $\leq 20/30$ was:

$$\begin{aligned} Q &= (TP + FP)/N \\ &= (104 + 188)/755 \\ &= 0.387 \\ &= p(T+) \end{aligned}$$

The negative sign rate (Q′) at this cut-off was:

$$\begin{aligned} Q' &= (FN + TN)/N \\ &= (10 + 453)/755 \\ &= 0.613 \\ &= 1 - Q \\ &= p(T-) \end{aligned}$$

Many of the measures derived from the 2×2 contingency table may be dependent on level of the test, Q, evident as variation with test cut-off. Looking at Q is one of the recommended steps in designing, conducting, reporting, and interpreting receiver operating characteristic (ROC) analyses to support clinical decision making ([30], p.205) (see Sect. 7.2).

Reading diagonally in Fig. 1.3, there are two diagonal ratios. The main diagonal (upper left to lower right) is given by:

$$R = (TP + TN)/N = (a + d)/N = r/N$$

The off diagonal (lower left to upper right) is given by:

$$R' = (1 - R) = (FP + FN)/N = (b + c)/N = r'/N$$
$$R + R' = 1$$

Using the nomenclature of sets, R' is the complement of R, and R and R' are disjoint sets.

R is sometimes known as "proportion correct" or "true rate" or accuracy (Acc; Sect. 3.2.5), and R' as "proportion incorrect" or "false rate" or misclassifications or error rate or inaccuracy (Inacc; Sect. 3.2.5).

Worked Examples: Proportions Correct and Incorrect (R, R')

In the screening test accuracy study of (MACE) [13], from the patient cohort (N = 755), at the MACE cut-off of ≤ 20/30, the test outcomes were as follows: TP = 104, FN = 10, FP = 188, and TN = 453.

Hence the proportion correct (R) at MACE cut-off ≤ 20/30 was:

$$
\begin{aligned}
R &= (TP + TN)/N \\
&= (104 + 453)/755 \\
&= 0.737
\end{aligned}
$$

The proportion incorrect (R') at this cut-off was:

$$
\begin{aligned}
R' &= (FP + FN)/N \\
&= (188 + 10)/755 \\
&= 0.263 \\
&= 1 - R
\end{aligned}
$$

Hereafter, Acc and Inacc will be used throughout this book, rather than R and R', to denote proportion correct and proportion incorrect respectively.

Many of the parameters derived from the 2×2 matrix and discussed in later chapters may be expressed in terms of P and Q (see, for example, Sects. 2.3.4, 2.3.5, 4.1, 4.2, 4.3, 4.4, 4.5, 4.8.1 and 4.8.3).

1.3.3   Pre-test Odds

Pre-test odds are given by the ratio of prevalence (or pre-test probability; Sect. 1.3.2) of instances with and without the item of interest (e.g. diagnosis, observation):

$$Pre - test\,odds\ = P/(1 - P)$$
$$= P/P'$$

In probability notation:

$$Pre - test\,odds\ =\ p(D+)/p(D-)$$

These are the odds favouring an event. Odds against the event are given by:

$$Pre - test\,odds\,against\ = (1 - P)/P$$
$$= P'/P$$

In probability notation:

$$Pre - test\,odds\ against\ =\ p(D-)/p(D+)$$

Worked Examples: Pre-test Odds for and Against

In the screening test accuracy study of (MACE) [13], in the total patient cohort ($N = 755$) the prevalence of dementia (P) was 0.151 and the prevalence of the absence of dementia ($1 - P$) was therefore 0.849 (Sect. 1.3.2).

Hence the pre-test odds of dementia were:

$$Pre - test\,odds = P/(1 - P)$$
$$= 0.151/0.849$$
$$= 0.178$$

The pre-test odds against dementia were:

$$Pre - test\,odds\,against = (1 - P)/P$$
$$= 0.849/0.151$$
$$= 5.62$$

The pre-test odds can be simply converted to pre-test probability:

$$Pre - test\,probability\ =\ Pre - test\,odds/(1 + Pre - test\,odds)$$

$$\text{Pre} - \text{test probability} = \quad 1/(1 + \text{Pre} - \text{test odds against})$$

Comparison of pre-test odds and post-test odds may be used in the Bayesian evaluation of tests (see Sect. 2.3.6). These odds also have a role in combining test results (Sects. 8.2.1 and 8.2.2).

1.4 Type I (α) and Type II (β) Errors

A variant of the simple 2×2 contingency table may be constructed which cross-classifies all instances (N) according to the outcome of the null hypothesis (Fig. 1.5), since this leads to a binary outcome (reject or do not reject). Here, the "true status" (vertical columns) refers to whether the null hypothesis is true or false, whilst the "test outcome" (horizontal rows) refers to whether or not the null hypothesis is rejected.

Type I (or α) error rate is the probability of rejecting the null hypothesis when in reality the null hypothesis is true; in other words, detecting an effect that does not exist (false positive), an error of commission.

Type II (or β) error rate, sometimes denoted power, is the probability of not rejecting the null hypothesis when it is in reality false (false negative); in other words, failing to detect an effect that does exist, an error of omission.

These terms may be rearranged, such that $1 - \beta$ is the probability of rejecting the null hypothesis when it is false, or $\beta = (1 - \text{power})$.

- Null hypothesis false, rejected (i.e. correct) $= 1 - \beta$ ("power")
- Null hypothesis true, rejected $= \alpha$ (false positive, type I error)
- Null hypothesis false, fail to reject $= \beta$ (false negative, type II error)
- Null hypothesis true, fail to reject (i.e. correct) $= 1 - \alpha$

		True Status	
		Null hypothesis false	**Null hypothesis true**
Test Outcome	**Reject null**	Correct: $1 - \beta$, power	Type I error: α, false positive
	Fail to reject null	Type II error: β, false negative	Correct: $1 - \alpha$

Fig. 1.5. 2×2 table using error notation

It should be noted that the four cells here are not equivalent to the four cells in the simple 2×2 table (Figs. 1.1 and 1.2). Henceforward the terms $1 - \beta$, α, β, and $1 - \alpha$ will be referred to as "error notation", and equations using this notation as "error equations".

Testing the null hypothesis by calculating p values is fraught with the possibility of drawing incorrect conclusions. The conventional tendency to "dichotomise" p values as significant or non-significant at the 0.05 level risks both type I ($p < 0.05$ may be a false positive) and type II ($p > 0.05$ may be a false negative) errors [2].

Type I (false positive) and type II (false negative) errors have also been characterised as related to the setting of epistemic thresholds: type I error is a manifestation of excessive belief and false knowledge, whereas type II error manifests excessive doubt and hence false ignorance ([9], p.71). The consequences of the setting of such epistemic thresholds are further considered in Sects. 2.3.6 and 3.2.4.

1.5   Calibration: Decision Thresholds or Cut-Offs

When constructing a 2×2 contingency table, test outcome may be obvious (e.g. a clinical sign is either present or absent, a forecast was either made or not made). Sometimes, however, the classification is not binary or categorical, for example when using tests with a quantitative range of scores or continuous values. Measurement scales may be classified in various ways, with one system distinguishing between those scales with variables in ordered categories the distances between which either have the same meaning (linear; interval data) or have different or unknown meaning (non-linear; ordinal data) [26]. Many scales used in clinical practice are ordinal in nature [18]. They may thereby run the risk of being subject to the fallacies noted by Stephen J. Gould (1941–2002): converting complex abstract concepts into single concrete entities, and ranking multiple complex variables into a single scale [8].

For the purposes of constructing a 2×2 contingency table using quantitative scales, there is a need to dichotomise results according to a chosen threshold, also variously known as a cut-off, cut-point, decision threshold, dichotomisation point, or positivity criterion. For some tests, cut-off point(s) may be specified, for example in the test manual or in the index publication. However, these may not be readily transferable to other study populations. Defining the optimal cut-off(s) may be achieved by various methods ([15], p.36–41, [19]) (see Sect. 7.3), although it has been argued that cut-offs should not be determined post hoc as this will risk introducing bias into study results [6]. This calibration process, the setting of the decision threshold(s) or cut-off(s), so that tests which produce continuous scale data may be used as if they were binary classifiers, will affect many of the outcome measures of a 2×2 contingency table. The setting of a cut-off will determine the level of the test, Q (Sect. 1.3.2).

The shortcomings of such dichotomisation are recognised: greater statistical power is afforded by the continuous approach [1, 5]. However, in clinical practice such dichotomisation is often pragmatic. Clinicians (and indeed patients) may generally be said to prefer binary classifiers (e.g. screen positive vs screen negative; target diagnosis present vs absent) since their categorical nature gives an impression of certainty and clarifies whether or not a medical intervention is applied. (An interesting illustration of the social ramifications of setting an arbitrary test threshold may be seen in Ursula Le Guin's short story entitled SQ, probably standing for Sanity Quotient, dating from 1978 ([20], p.359–70)).

1.6 Uncertain or Inconclusive Test Results

There are potential problems with the use of dichotomous thresholds. Things which once appeared or were conceptualised as binary or dimorphic may prove to be part of a spectrum or continuum (e.g. consciousness, sexuality). Disease entities once codified as binary may subsequently be recognised as spectrum disorders (e.g. Alzheimer's disease, compare diagnostic criteria of 1984 [22] and 2014 [7]). Providing a single cut-off score may therefore risk misclassification. Indeed, some authors advocate the abandonment of binary disease categories in favour of a probability dysfunction model based on risk of harm according to risk banding [4].

Three-way classification, or trichotomisation, has been suggested as a method to allow better classification accuracy but at the cost of not classifying a proportion of cases. Specifically, uncertain test scores, the most error-prone, are excluded or deselected from classification. This may be a substantial proportion of the test cohort, particularly if the test has limited strength, with unclassified individuals requiring further assessment for correct classification, achieved either by watchful waiting/active surveillance or by the application of further (more sophisticated, more expensive, more risky) tests [12].

Higher order contingency tables (2 × 3, 2 × 4, 3 × 3) may also be a method to address problems of this kind (Sect. 8.5.1).

1.7 Measures Derived from a 2 × 2 Contingency Table; Confidence Intervals

Aside from the marginal totals and probabilities (Sect. 1.3), a large number of other measures may be derived from a 2 × 2 contingency table. Many of these measures will be described in the subsequent chapters of this book, including but not limited to sensitivity and specificity, predictive values, and likelihood ratios. None is perfect, all have potential shortcomings, as well as utilities, in describing the outcomes of a contingency table. Indeed, it might be intuited that the very multiplicity of these measures suggests their inadequacy: all summary statistics reduce the information to a single characteristic of the data. (Perhaps a vector in the unit 4-dimensional space of a hypercube or tesseract might be a unique outcome descriptor for each 2 × 2 table, and be a potential comparator measure, but whether this would prove readily applicable, particularly in clinical practice, is highly questionable.) These measures permit an approximate generalisation to be substituted for an absolute rule (except in limit cases where the absolute rule holds).

To account for sampling variability, calculation of confidence intervals (or compatibility intervals [2]) for each point estimate is recommended as a measure of precision. This quantification of statistical uncertainty is typically expressed using the 95% confidence interval (95% CI), in other words one can be 95% certain that the true value lies between these limits. Narrow confidence intervals (greater precision) result from large sample sizes, whereas small sample sizes may be associated with broad confidence intervals (lesser precision, hence more often give extreme results) [28]. Failure to quote confidence intervals may influence the generalizability of diagnostic studies ([15], p.53–4).

Confidence intervals may be calculated in various ways. For simple estimates, 95% confidence intervals (e.g. for sensitivity, specificity, predictive values; Chap. 2) may be calculated as:

$$p + / - 1.96\sqrt{p \cdot (1-p)/n}$$

A log method is used to calculate confidence intervals for measures such as likelihood ratios (Sect. 2.3.5), diagnostic odds ratio (Sect. 2.4.1) and the Efficiency Index (Sect. 5.11). For receiver operating characteristic (ROC) curves the standard error of the area under the curve is calculated (Sect. 7.2.2).

Worked examples: Confidence intervals for P, Q, and R (or Acc)

In the screening test accuracy study of (MACE) [13], in the total patient cohort (N = 755) the prevalence of dementia (P) was 0.151 and the prevalence of the absence of dementia (1 − P) was therefore 0.849 (Sect. 1.3.2).
Hence the 95% confidence intervals (95% CI) for P are:

$$95\% \, CI = 1.96\sqrt{p \cdot (1-p)/n}$$
$$= 0.151 + / - 1.96\sqrt{0.151.(1-0.151)/755}$$
$$= 0.151 + / - 0.0255$$
$$P = 0.151(95\% \, CI = 0.125 - 0.176)$$

In the same study, the positive sign rate (Q) was 0.387 and the negative sign rate (1 − Q) was 0.613 (Sect. 1.3.2).
Hence the 95% confidence intervals (95% CI) for Q are:

$$95\% \, CI = 1.96\sqrt{p \cdot (1-p)/n}$$
$$= 0.387 + / - 1.96\sqrt{0.387 \cdot (1-0.387)/755}$$

$$= 0.387 + /-0.0177$$
$$Q = 0.151(95\% \text{ CI} = 0.369 - 0.404)$$

In the same study, the fraction correct (R) or accuracy (Acc) was 0.737 and the fraction incorrect (1 − R) or inaccuracy (Inacc) was 0.263 (Sect. 1.3.2). Hence the 95% confidence intervals (95% CI) for R are:

$$95\% \text{ CI} = 1.96\sqrt{p \cdot (1-p)/n}$$
$$= 0.737 + /-1.96\sqrt{0.737.(1-0.737)/755}$$
$$= 0.737 + /-0.0160$$
$$R = 0.737 \,(95\% \text{ CI} = 0.722 - 0.754)$$

Note the narrow confidence intervals for each of these point estimates.

References

1. Altman DG, Royston P. The cost of dichotomising continuous variables. BMJ. 2006;332:1080.
2. Amrhein V, Greenland S, McShane B. Scientists rise up against statistical significance. Nature. 2019;567:305–7.
3. Ares J, Lara J, Lizcano D, Martinez MA. Who discovered the binary system and arithmetic? Did Leibniz plagiarize Caramuel? Sci Eng Ethics. 2018;24:173–88.
4. Baum ML. The neuroethics of biomarkers. What the development of bioprediction means for moral responsibility, justice, and the nature of mental disorder. Oxford; Oxford University Press; 2016.
5. Cohen J. The cost of dichotomization. Appl Psychol Meas. 1983;7:249–53.
6. Davis DH, Creavin ST, Noel-Storr A et al. Neuropsychological tests for the diagnosis of Alzheimer's disease dementia and other dementias: a generic protocol for cross-sectional and delayed-verification studies. Cochrane Database Syst Rev. 2013;3:CD010460.
7. Dubois B, Feldman HH, Jacova C et al. Advancing research diagnostic criteria for Alzheimer's disease: the IWG-2 criteria. Lancet Neurol. 2014;13:614–29 [Erratum Lancet Neurol. 2014;13:757].
8. Gould SJ. The mismeasure of man. New York: Norton; 1981.
9. Han PKJ. Uncertainty in medicine. A framework for tolerance. Oxford: Oxford University Press; 2021.
10. Hsieh S, McGrory S, Leslie F, Dawson K, Ahmed S, Butler CR, et al. The Mini-Addenbrooke's Cognitive Examination: a new assessment tool for dementia. Dement Geriatr Cogn Disord. 2015;39:1–11.
11. Kraemer HC. Evaluating medical tests. Objective and quantitative guidelines. Newbery Park, California: Sage; 1992.
12. Landsheer JA. The clinical relevance of methods for handling inconclusive medical test results: quantification of uncertainty in medical decision-making and screening. Diagnostics (Basel). 2018;8:32.
13. Larner AJ. MACE for diagnosis of dementia and MCI: examining cut-offs and predictive values. Diagnostics (Basel). 2019;9:E51.

14. Larner AJ. Applying Kraemer's Q (positive sign rate): some implications for diagnostic test accuracy study results. Dement Geriatr Cogn Dis Extra. 2019;9:389–96.
15. Larner AJ. Diagnostic test accuracy studies in dementia. A pragmatic approach. 2nd edition. London: Springer; 2019.
16. Larner AJ. The "attended alone" and "attended with" signs in the assessment of cognitive impairment: a revalidation. Postgrad Med. 2020;132:595–600.
17. Larner AJ. Mini-Addenbrooke's Cognitive Examination (MACE): a useful cognitive screening instrument in older people? Can Geriatr J. 2020;23:199–204.
18. Larner AJ. Manual of screeners for dementia. Pragmatic test accuracy studies. London: Springer; 2020.
19. Larner AJ. Defining "optimal" test cut-off using global test metrics: evidence from a cognitive screening instrument. Neurodegener Dis Manag. 2020;10:223–30.
20. Le Guin UK. The wind's twelve quarters & The compass rose. London: Gollancz; 2015.
21. Matthews JR. Quantification and the quest for medical certainty. Princeton: Princeton University Press; 1995.
22. McKhann G, Drachman D, Folstein M, Katzman R, Price D, Stadlan EM. Clinical diagnosis of Alzheimer's disease. Report of the NINCDS-ADRDA work group under the auspices of the Department of Health and Human Service Task forces on Alzheimer's disease. Neurology. 1984;34:939–44.
23. McNicol D. A primer of signal detection theory. Mahwah, New Jersey and London: Lawrence Erlbaum Associates; 2005.
24. Pearson K. Draper's Company Research Memoirs. Biometric Series I. Mathematical contributions to the theory of evolution XIII. On the theory of contingency and its relation to association and normal correlation. London: Dulau & Co.; 1904.
25. Porter TM. Karl Pearson. The scientific life in a statistical age. Princeton and Oxford: Princeton University Press; 2004.
26. Stevens SS. On the theory of scales of measurement. Science. 1946;103:677–80.
27. Stigler S. The missing early history of contingency tables. Ann Fac Sci Toulouse. 2002;11:563–73.
28. Tan SH, Tan SB. The correct interpretation of confidence intervals. Proceedings of Singapore Healthcare. 2010;19:276–8.
29. Wojtowicz A, Larner AJ. Diagnostic test accuracy of cognitive screeners in older people. Prog Neurol Psychiatry. 2017;21(1):17–21.
30. Youngstrom EA. A primer on receiver operating characteristic analysis and diagnostic efficiency statistics for pediatric psychology: we are ready to ROC. J Pediatr Psychol. 2014;39:204–21.

Chapter 2
Paired Measures

Contents

2.1 Introduction

Several paired measures may be derived from the basic 2×2 contingency table (described in Chap. 1). The classification of these measures as error-based, information-based, and association-based, following Bossuyt [2], is used in this chapter. Other classifications might have been used, such as test-oriented measures (e.g. sensitivity and specificity, false positive and false negative rates, likelihood ratios) versus patient-oriented measures (predictive values, predictive ratios).

2.2 Error-Based Measures

2.2.1 Sensitivity (Sens) and Specificity (Spec), or True Positive and True Negative Rates (TPR, TNR)

Yerushalmy [43] and Neyman [35] are usually credited as the first authors to discuss the statistical aspects of screening and diagnostic tests. Yerushalmy, assessing radiological methods, introduced the terms sensitivity (Sens) and specificity (Spec) to denote respectively the inherent ability of a test to detect correctly a condition when it is present (in the terms of signal detection theory a "hit") and to rule it out correctly when it is absent ("correct rejection").

Sens and Spec are conditional probabilities with range from 0 to 1, with higher values better. They are "uncalibrated measures of test quality … with a variable zero-point and scale" ([16], p.65). There is a trade-off between Sens and Spec, since as the value of one rises the other falls.

Sensitivity (Sens) is sometimes known as true positive rate or ratio (TPR), hit rate, recall, or success ratio. In medical practice it is the probability of a positive test result given the presence of disease, or the proportion of test positivity in the presence of a target condition, hence more generally a positive classification by the test in the presence of a given class.

In literal notation (Fig. 2.1):

$$Sens = TP/(TP + FN)$$

or, with marginal total notation:

$$Sens = TP/p$$

In algebraic notation:

$$Sens = a/(a + c)$$
$$= a/p$$

In error notation (see Fig. 1.5):

$$Sens = (1 - \beta)$$

Sens may also be expressed in probability notation. If a test may be either positive, T+, or negative, T−, when used to distinguish between the presence, D+, or absence, D−, of a target disease, then:

$$Sens = p(T + | D+)$$

		True Status		
		Condition present (= case)	**Condition absent (= non case)**	r '
Test Outcome	**Positive**	True positive [TP] (a)	False positive [FP] (b)	q
	Negative	False negative [FN] (c)	True negative [TN] (d)	q '
		p	p '	r

Paired measures (algebraic notation only):

Sens (TPR)	=	a/(a + c)		
Spec (TNR)	=	d/(b + d)		
FPR	=	(1 − Spec)	=	b/(b + d)
FNR	=	(1 − Sens)	=	c/(a + c)
PPV	=	a/(a + b)		
NPV	=	d/(c + d)		
FDR	=	(1 − PPV)	=	b/(a + b)
FRR	=	(1 − NPV)	=	c/(c + d)
PLR	=	TPR/(1 − TNR)	=	[a/(a + c)]/[b/(b + d)]
NLR	=	(1 − TPR)/TNR	=	[c/(a + c)]/[d/(b + d)]
DOR	=	ad/bc =	PLR/NLR	
EOR	=	ab/cd		
PCUI	=	Sens x PPV	=	a/(a + c) x a/(a + b)
NCUI	=	Spec x NPV	=	d/(b + d) x d/(c + d)
PCDI	=	FNR x FDR	=	c/(a + c) x b/(a + b)
NCDI	=	FPR x FRR	=	b/(b + d) x c/(c + d)

Fig. 2.1 2 × 2 contingency table with literal and algebraic notation, marginal totals, and derived paired measures

Specificity (Spec) is sometimes known as true negative rate or ratio (TNR). In medical practice it is the probability of a negative test result given the absence of disease, or the proportion of test negativity among the healthy, hence more generally a negative classification by the test in the absence of a given class. Hence both Sens and Spec are test-oriented measures.

In literal notation:

$$\text{Spec} = \text{TN}/(\text{FP} + \text{TN})$$

or, with marginal total notation:

$$\text{Spec} = \text{TN}/p'$$

In algebraic notation:

$$\text{Spec} = d/(b + d)$$
$$= d/p'$$

In error notation (see Fig. 1.5):

$$\text{Spec} = (1 - \alpha)$$

In probability notation:

$$\text{Spec} = p(\,T-\,|\,D-\,)$$

Worked Examples: Sens, Spec

The Mini-Addenbrooke's Cognitive Examination (MACE) [12] was subjected to a screening test accuracy study in a large patient cohort, $N = 755$ [17]. At the MACE cut-off of $\leq 20/30$, the test outcomes for the diagnosis of dementia were (as shown in the 2×2 contingency table, Fig. 2.2): $TP = 104$, $FN = 10$, $FP = 188$, and $TN = 453$.

		Diagnosis	
		Dementia present	**Dementia absent**
MACE Outcome	**≤20/30**	True positive [TP] = **104**	False positive [FP] = **188**
	>20/30	False negative [FN] = **10**	True negative [TN] = **453**

Fig. 2.2 2×2 contingency table for Mini-Addenbrooke's cognitive examination (MACE) outcomes ($N = 755$) for the diagnosis of dementia at MACE cut-off of $\leq 20/30$ (data from [17])

Hence the values for Sens and Spec at this cut-off are:

$$\text{Sens} = \text{TP}/(\text{TP} + \text{FN})$$
$$= 104/(104 + 10)$$

$$= 0.912$$

$$\text{Spec} = \text{TN}/(\text{FP} + \text{TN})$$
$$= 453/(188 + 453)$$
$$= 0.707$$

Sens and Spec were once thought to be invariant, intrinsic test properties, independent of study sample and location. Certainly they are algebraically unrelated to the base rate, P (Sect. 1.3.2), and hence insensitive to changes in class distribution, being strict columnar ratios. However, in medical practice it is now recognised that heterogeneity of clinical populations (spectrum bias) imposes potentially serious limitations on the utility of Sens and Spec measures, since very different values may be found, for example in different patient subgroups within the sampled population, i.e. Sens and Spec are not independent of disease prevalence [3, 11, 28, 29] (Sect. 3.4).

Worked Example: Effect of Disease Prevalence on Sens, Spec

In the aforementioned study of MACE [17], test performance was analysed in patient cohorts aged ≥ 65 years (n = 287) and ≥ 75 years (n = 119), in whom the prevalence of cognitive impairment (dementia and mild cognitive impairment) was anticipated to be higher than in the whole cohort, since the prevalence of dementia increases with age. The table shows Sens and Spec for cognitive impairment at the MACE cut-off of $\leq 25/30$ (with 95% confidence intervals) in the different cohorts.

Cohort	Whole	≥ 65 years	≥ 75 years
N	755	287	119
Prevalence of cognitive impairment	0.445	0.749	0.933
Sens	0.967 (0.948–0.986)	0.963 (0.937–0.988)	0.991 (0.973–1.00)
Spec	0.458 (0.411–0.506)	0.528 (0.412–0.643)	0.375 (0.040–0.710)

Hence this analysis clearly illustrates the different values for Sens and Spec in subgroups with different disease prevalence (or pre-test probability) [20]. A similar analysis has been performed for the Free-Cog screening instrument and the original MACE analysis has been extended to examine 5-year age cohorts between the ages of 50 and 79 [26].

Sens and Spec also vary with test cut-off [17] or Q [18], prompting the development of the "quality measures" [27] (explored in depth in Chap. 6), QSens and QSpec (Sect. 6.2.1).

2.2.2 False Positive Rate (FPR), False Negative Rate (FNR)

False positive and false negative rates denote respectively the inherent capacity or propensity of a test to detect incorrectly a condition when it is absent (in the terms of signal detection theory a "false alarm" or "false hit") and not to detect it correctly when it is present (a "miss"). Like Sens and Spec, false positive and false negative rates are conditional probabilities with range from 0 to 1.

False positive rate or ratio (FPR) is a measure of incorrect classification. In medical practice this is the probability of the test result classifying non-cases as cases, and more generally of classifying non-events as events ("overcalls"). FPR ranges from 0 to 1, with lower values better.

FPR is sometimes known as the "false alarm rate" but this latter terminology is not used here because of possible confusion with another parameter for which this term may also be used which is also known as the false discovery rate (see Sect. 2.3.2). The term "fall out" is also sometimes used to denote FPR.

In literal notation (Fig. 2.1):

$$FPR = FP/(FP + TN)$$

or, with marginal total notation:

$$FPR = FP/p'$$

In algebraic notation:

$$FPR = b/(b + d)$$
$$= b/p'$$

In error notation (see Fig. 1.5):

$$FPR = \alpha$$

In probability notation:

$$FPR = p(\, T + \mid D- \,)$$

FPR is analogous to Type I or α error (Sect. 1.5). FPR is the complement of specificity (see Sect. 3.2.2).

False negative rate or ratio (FNR), or miss rate, is another measure of incorrect classification. In medical practice it is the probability of the test result classifying cases as non-cases, and more generally of classifying events or instances as non-events or non-instances ("undercalls"). FNR ranges from 0 to 1, with lower values better.

In literal notation (Fig. 2.1):

$$FNR = FN/(FN + TP)$$

or, with marginal total notation:

$$FNR = FN/p$$

In algebraic notation:

$$FNR = c/(a + c)$$
$$= c/p$$

In error notation (see Fig. 1.5):

$$FNR = \beta$$

In probability notation:

$$FNR = p(\,T - \,|\,D+\,)$$

FNR is analogous to Type II or β error (Sect. 1.5). FNR is the complement of sensitivity (see Sect. 3.2.1).

Worked Examples: FPR, FNR

In a screening test accuracy study of MACE [17], at the MACE cut-off of ≤ 20/30, the test outcomes were as follows (Fig. 2.2): TP = 104, FN = 10, FP = 188, and TN = 453.

Hence the values for FPR and FNR at this cut-off are:

$$FPR = FP/(FP + TN)$$
$$= 188/(188 + 453)$$
$$= 0.293$$

$$FNR = FN/(FN + TP)$$
$$= 10/(10 + 104)$$
$$= 0.088$$

Like Sens and Spec, FPR and FNR are strict columnar ratios and hence algebraically are unrelated to the base rate, P, and hence are at least notionally insensitive to changes in class distribution. However, as with Sens and Spec, values may vary with the heterogeneity of clinical populations (spectrum bias).

FPR and FNR vary with test cut-off [17] or Q [18], prompting the development of the "quality measures," QFPR and QFNR (Sect. 6.2.2).

The appropriate balance between FP and FN in any test, or their relative costs, may need to be factored into clinical judgments (see Sect. 3.2.4 for further discussion). Of note, many measures assume these costs to be equal (e.g. diagnostic odds ratio, Sect. 2.4.1; accuracy, Sect. 3.2.5; Youden index, Sect. 4.2) but this is often not the case in clinical practice.

2.3   Information-Based Measures

2.3.1   Positive and Negative Predictive Values (PPV, NPV)

Predictive values give the probability that a disease is present or absent given the test is positive or negative, or more generally that the test will forecast the correct outcome or classification [1]. Predictive values range from 0 to 1, with higher values better. Predictive values are calculated using values from both columns of the 2 × 2 contingency table (cf. Sens and Spec; Sect. 2.2.1), hence are sensitive to class imbalance or skews, or in other words are dependent on disease prevalence,

Positive predictive value (PPV) is the probability of disease in a patient given a positive test, also known as the post-positive test probability of disease, or post-test probability, or precision (see Sect. 7.4.2). In the weather forecasting literature, the term "probability of detection" (POD) or prefigurance is sometimes used [40].

In literal notation (Fig. 2.1):

$$PPV = TP/(TP + FP)$$

or, with marginal total notation:

$$PPV = TP/q$$

In algebraic notation:

$$PPV = a/(a+b)$$
$$= a/q$$

In probability notation:

$$PPV = p(D+ \mid T+)$$

Negative predictive value (NPV) is the probability of the absence of disease in a patient given a negative test, hence also known as the post-negative test probability of absence of disease. Hence both PPV and NPV may be described as patient-oriented measures (cf. Sens and Spec as test-oriented measures).

In literal notation (Fig. 2.1):

$$NPV = TN/(FN + TN)$$

or, with marginal total notation:

$$NPV = TN/q'$$

In algebraic notation:

$$NPV = d/(c+d)$$
$$= d/q'$$

In probability notation:

$$NPV = p(D- \mid T-)$$

Worked Examples: PPV, NPV

In a screening test accuracy study of MACE [17], at the MACE cut-off of $\leq$ 20/30, the test outcomes were as follows (Fig. 2.2): TP = 104, FN = 10, FP = 188, and TN = 453.

Hence the raw, unadjusted, predictive values at this cut-off are:

$$PPV = TP/(TP + FP)$$
$$= 104/(104 + 188)$$
$$= 0.356$$

$$NPV = TN/(FN + TN)$$
$$= 453/(10 + 453)$$
$$= 0.978$$

Predictive values are scalar values based on information from both columns of the 2×2 table (cf. Sens and Spec). Hence, they vary with prevalence, P (Sect. 2.3.4), and are sensitive to class imbalance, for which reason their values may be described as "unstable" and do not necessarily travel well from one situation to another [44].

Predictive values also vary with the level of the test, Q, for which reason "quality measures," QPPV and QNPV, may be used (Sect. 6.3.1).

2.3.2 False Discovery Rate (FDR), False Reassurance Rate (FRR)

The false discovery rate (FDR) is a measure of the probability of the absence of disease given an abnormal test (i.e. identifying a non-case as a case), hence also known as the post-positive test probability of absence of disease. FDR ranges from 0 to 1, with lower values better.

FDR has sometimes been known as the false alarm rate. "False alarm rate" is potentially an ambiguous term: it has also been used on occasion to mean both the false positive rate (FPR) (e.g. [16], p.64) and the false negative rate (FNR) [38] (Sect. 2.2.2). Hence the FDR terminology is preferred here in order to avoid any possible confusion.

In literal notation (Fig. 2.1):

$$FDR = FP/(TP + FP)$$

or, with marginal total notation:

$$FDR = FP/q$$

In algebraic notation:

$$FDR = b/(a + b)$$
$$= b/q$$

FDR is the complement of PPV (see Sect. 3.3.1):

$$FDR = 1 - PPV$$

In probability notation:

$$FDR = p(D - | T+)$$

False reassurance rate (FRR), sometimes known as false omission rate (FOR), is a measure of the probability of the presence of disease given a normal test (i.e. identifying a case as a non-case), hence also known as the post-negative test probability of disease. FRR ranges from 0 to 1, with lower values better.

In literal notation (Fig. 2.1):

$$FRR = FN/(FN + TN)$$

or, with marginal total notation:

$$FRR = FN/q'$$

In algebraic notation:

$$FRR = c/(c + d)$$
$$= c/q'$$

FRR is the complement of NPV (see Sect. 3.3.2):

$$FRR = 1 - NPV$$

In probability notation:

$$FRR = p(D + | T-)$$

Worked Examples: FDR, FRR

In a screening test accuracy study of MACE [17], at the MACE cut-off of $\leq$ 20/30 (Fig. 2.2), TP = 104, FN = 10, FP = 188, and TN = 453.

Hence the values for FDR and FRR are:

$$FDR = FP/(TP + FP)$$
$$= 188/(104 + 188)$$
$$= 0.644$$

$$FRR = FN/(FN + TN)$$
$$= 10/(10 + 453)$$
$$= 0.022$$

FDR and FRR vary with the level of the test, Q, for which reason "quality measures," QFDR and QFRR, may be used (Sect. 6.3.2).

2.3.3 Bayes' Formula; Standardized Positive and Negative Predictive Values (SPPV, SNPV)

It is possible to calculate PPV and NPV at any disease prevalence based on values for Sens and Spec since the latter are (relatively) resistant to changes in prevalence (although not immutably fixed; Sect. 2.2.1). This approach to probability revision is given by Bayes' formula, after Thomas Bayes (1702–61), hence [1]:

$$PPV = Sens \times P/(Sens \times P) + [(1 - Spec) \times (1 - P)]$$
$$= Sens \times P/(Sens \times P) + [FPR \times (1 - P)]$$

$$NPV = Spec \times (1 - P)/[Spec \times (1 - P)] + [(1 - Sens) \times P]$$
$$= Spec \times (1 - P)/[Spec \times (1 - P)] + [FNR \times P]$$

This may be expressed in probability notation as:

$$PPV = p(T+ \mid D+) \cdot p(D+)/p(T+ \mid D+) \cdot p(D+) + p(T+ \mid D-) \cdot p(D-)$$

$$NPV = p(T- \mid D+) \cdot p(D-)/p(T- \mid D-) \cdot p(D-) + p(T- \mid D+) \cdot p(D+)$$

Heston [9, 10] defined "standardized predictive values" as the predictive values calculated at 50% disease prevalence (i.e. $P = P' = 0.5$, a balanced class distribution, or no class imbalance; Sect. 1.3.2). Hence, using Bayes' formula:

$$SPPV = 0.5 \times Sens/(0.5 \times Sens) + [0.5 \times (1 - Spec)]$$
$$= 0.5 \times Sens/(0.5 \times Sens) + (0.5 \times FPR)$$

$$SNPV = 0.5 \times Spec/(0.5 \times Spec) + [0.5 \times (1 - Sens)]$$
$$= 0.5 \times Spec/(0.5 \times Spec) + (0.5 \times FNR)$$

Heston also suggested the potential clinical value of performing predictive value calculations for prevalence rates of 25% and 75%. Estimates of standardized predictive values, SPPV and SNPV, may differ from PPV and NPV, the differences being larger when prevalence deviates more strongly from 0.5.

Worked Examples: SPPV, SNPV

In a screening test accuracy study of the MACE [17], at the MACE cut-off $\leq$ 20/30 (Fig. 2.2), Sens = 0.912 and Spec = 0.707 (see Sect. 2.2.1). Dementia prevalence in the patient cohort (N = 755) was 0.151 (Sect. 1.3.2).

For a dementia prevalence of 0.5, the standardized predictive values are:

$$\text{SPPV} = 0.5 \times \text{Sens}/(0.5 \times \text{Sens}) + [0.5 \times (1 - \text{Spec})]$$
$$= 0.5 \times 0.912/(0.5 \times 0.912) + [0.5 \times (1 - 0.707)]$$
$$= 0.757$$

$$\text{SNPV} = 0.5 \times \text{Spec}/[0.5 \times \text{Spec}] + [0.5 \times (1 - \text{Sens})]$$
$$= 0.5 \times 0.707/[0.5 \times 0.707] + [0.5 \times (1 - 0.912)]$$
$$= 0.889$$

Comparing the SPPV and SNPV values with PPV and NPV (Sect. 2.3.1), SPPV is much better than PPV (0.757 vs 0.356), whilst SNPV is a little worse than NPV (0.889 vs 0.978).

This possibility for rescaling PPV and NPV for different values of P is sometimes exploited by researchers to give an indication of test performance in settings other than that of their own study. Examples amongst cognitive screening tests include the Addenbrooke's Cognitive Examination [31], the Addenbrooke's Cognitive Examination Revised [33], and the Mini-Addenbrooke's Cognitive Examination [17], with PPV and NPV calculated at prevalence rates of 0.05, 0.1, 0.2, and 0.4. Indeed, PPV may be calculated across the complete range of prevalence or pre-test probabilities to produce a conditional probability plot (Sect. 2.3.7).

It is also possible to express FDR and FRR in probability notation. By Bayes' equation:

$$\text{FDR} = p(T + | D-) \cdot p(D-)/p(T + | D-) \cdot p(D-) + p(T + | D+) \cdot p(D+)$$
$$\text{FRR} = p(T - | D+) \cdot p(D+)/p(T - | D+) \cdot p(D+) + p(T - | D-) \cdot p(D-)$$

2.3.4   Interrelations of Sens, Spec, PPV, NPV, P, and Q

Sens, Spec, PPV, NPV, P, Q, and their complements, FNR, FPR, FDR, FRR, P' and Q', are all interrelated.

P and its complement P' (Sect. 1.3.2) may be expressed in terms of PPV, NPV, Q, and their respective complements:

$$P = PPV \cdot Q + (1 - NPV) \cdot Q'$$
$$= PPV \cdot Q + FRR.Q'$$

$$P' = (1 - PPV) \cdot Q + NPV \cdot Q'$$
$$= FDR \cdot Q + NPV \cdot Q'$$

Worked Examples: P and P' in Terms of PPV, NPV, and Q

In a screening test accuracy study of MACE [17], at the cut-off of $\leq 20/30$ where Q = 0.387 (Sect. 1.3.2), PPV = 0.356 and NPV = 0.978.

Hence the values for P and P' at this cut-off are:

$$P = PPV \cdot Q + (1 - NPV) \cdot Q'$$
$$= 0.138 + 0.013$$
$$= 0.151$$

$$P' = (1 - PPV) \cdot Q + NPV \cdot Q'$$
$$= 0.249 + 0.600$$
$$= 0.849$$

These values for P and P' are the same as those calculated from the base data in Sect. 1.3.2.

Q and its complement Q' may be expressed in terms of Sens, Spec, P, and their respective complements:

$$Q = Sens \cdot P + (1 - Spec) \cdot P'$$
$$= Sens \cdot P + FPR \cdot P'.$$

$$Q' = (1 - Sens) \cdot P + Spec \cdot P'$$
$$= FNR \cdot P + Spec \cdot P'$$

Worked Examples: Q and Q′ in Terms of Sens, Spec, and P

In a screening test accuracy study of MACE [17], at the cut-off of $\leq 20/30$ where $P = 0.151$, Sens $= 0.912$ and Spec $= 0.707$ (Sect. 2.2.1).

Hence the values for Q and Q′ at this cut-off are:

$$Q = \text{Sens} \cdot P + (1 - \text{Spec}) \cdot P'$$
$$= 0.138 + 0.249$$
$$= 0.387$$

$$Q' = (1 - \text{Sens}) \cdot P + \text{Spec} \cdot P'$$
$$= 0.013 + 0.600$$
$$= 0.613$$

These values for Q and Q′ are the same as those calculated from the base data in Sect. 1.3.2.

Sens and Spec may be expressed in terms of PPV, NPV, P, Q and their respective complements:

$$\text{Sens} = \text{PPV} \cdot Q/(\text{PPV} \cdot Q) + (1 - \text{NPV}) \cdot Q'$$
$$= \text{PPV} \cdot Q/(\text{PPV} \cdot Q) + (\text{FRR} \cdot Q')$$
$$= \text{PPV} \cdot Q/P$$

$$\text{Spec} = \text{NPV} \cdot Q'/(1 - \text{PPV}) \cdot Q + (\text{NPV} \cdot Q')$$
$$= \text{NPV} \cdot Q'/(\text{FDR} \cdot P) + (\text{NPV} \cdot Q')$$
$$= \text{NPV} \cdot Q'/P'$$

Worked Examples: Sens and Spec in Terms of PPV, NPV, P, and Q

In a screening test accuracy study of MACE [17], at the cut-off of $\leq 20/30$, PPV $= 0.356$, NPV $= 0.978$, P $= 0.151$, and Q $= 0.387$.

Hence the values for Sens and Spec at this cut-off are:

$$\text{Sens} = \text{PPV} \cdot Q/P$$
$$= 0.138/0.151$$
$$= 0.912$$

$$\text{Spec} = \text{NPV} \cdot Q'/P'$$
$$= 0.600/0.849$$
$$= 0.707$$

Values for Sens and Spec are the same as those calculated from the base data in Sect. 2.2.1.

PPV and NPV may be expressed in terms of Sens, Spec, P, Q and their respective complements (further developing the formulae in Sect. 2.3.3):

$$\text{PPV} = \text{Sens} \cdot P/(\text{Sens} \cdot P) + (1 - \text{Spec}) \cdot P'$$
$$= \text{Sens} \cdot P/(\text{Sens} \cdot P) + (\text{FPR} \cdot P')$$
$$= \text{Sens} \cdot P/Q$$

$$\text{NPV} = \text{Spec} \cdot P'/(1 - \text{Sens}) \cdot P + (\text{Spec} \cdot P')$$
$$= \text{Spec} \cdot P'/(\text{FNR} \cdot P) + (\text{Spec} \cdot P')$$
$$= (\text{Spec} \cdot P'/Q')$$

Worked Examples: PPV and NPV in Terms of Sens, Spec, P, and Q

In a screening test accuracy study of MACE [17], at the cut-off of $\leq 20/30$, Sens = 0.912, Spec = 0.707, P = 0.151, and Q = 0.387.

Hence the values for PPV and NPV at this cut-off are:

$$\text{PPV} = \text{Sens} \cdot P/Q$$
$$= 0.138/0.387$$
$$= 0.356$$

$$\text{NPV} = \text{Spec} \cdot P'/Q'$$
$$= 0.600/0.613$$
$$= 0.978$$

Values for PPV and NPV are the same as those calculated from the base data in Sect. 2.3.1.

A graphical method of presentation illustrating Sens, Spec, PPV, and NPV has been described, in which the distribution of affected and unaffected individuals is displayed respectively above and below a horizontal axis extending from normal to abnormal, with a vertical axis denoting the (potentially movable) test threshold. The different measures may be conceptually more easily appreciated using this diagrammatic approach (test accuracy and inaccuracy, Sect. 3.2.5, may also be shown in this way) [4].

2.3.5 Positive and Negative Likelihood Ratios (PLR, NLR)

First introduced into medical test evaluation in the mid-1970s [37, 41], likelihood ratios (LRs), also sometimes known as diagnostic likelihood ratios (DLRs), measure the change in pre-test odds (Sect. 1.3.3) to post-test odds (Sect. 2.3.6), and hence may be characterised as measures of probability revision based on Bayes' formula, or measures of diagnostic gain. They combine information about sensitivity and specificity [38] and hence are closely related to these terms.

The positive likelihood ratio (PLR; also sometimes denoted LR+) gives the odds of a positive test result in an affected individual relative to an unaffected:

$$PLR = Sens/(1 - Spec)$$
$$= Sens/FPR$$
$$= TPR/FPR$$

In literal notation:

$$PLR = [TP/(TP + FN)]/[FP/(FP + TN)]$$
$$= [TP/p]/[FP/p']$$
$$= [TP \cdot p']/[FP \cdot p]$$

In algebraic notation:

$$PLR = [a/(a + c)]/[b/(b + d)]$$
$$= [a \cdot (b + d)]/[b \cdot (a + c)]$$
$$= [a \cdot p']/[b \cdot p]$$

In error notation:

$$PLR = (1 - \beta)/\alpha$$

PLR can also be expressed in probability notation:

$$PLR = TPR/FPR$$
$$= p(T + | D+)/p(T + | D-)$$

The negative likelihood ratio (NLR; also sometimes denoted LR−) gives the odds of a negative test result in an affected individual relative to an unaffected.

$$NLR = (1 - Sens)/Spec$$
$$= FNR/Spec$$
$$= FNR/TNR$$

In literal notation:

$$NLR = [FN/(TP + FN)]/[TN/(FP + TN)]$$
$$= [FN/p]/[TN/p']$$
$$= [FN \cdot p']/[TN \cdot p]$$

In algebraic notation:

$$NLR = [c/(a + c)]/[d/(b + d)]$$
$$= [c \cdot (b + d)]/[d \cdot (a + c)]$$
$$= [c \cdot p']/[d \cdot p]$$

In error notation:

$$NLR = \beta/(1 - \alpha)$$

NLR can also be expressed in probability notation:

$$NLR = FNR/TNR$$
$$= p(T - | D+)/p(T - | D-)$$

More generally, if the outcome of a test is R_i, then:

$$LR = p(R_i | D+)/p(R_i | D-)$$

Likelihood ratios may be qualitatively classified according to their distance from 1, denoting a useless test, to indicate the change in probability of disease (Table 2.1, left hand column) [14]; for PLR end points range from 1 to ∞; for NLR they range from 0 to 1.

A distinction may be drawn between result-specific and category-specific LRs ([13], p.175). A result-specific LR refers to the ratio of the probability of observing that result conditional on the presence of the target (disease, diagnosis) to the probability of observing that result conditional on the absence of the target. However, more often in clinical practice dichotomised test results are cumulated to produce a category-specific LR.

Table 2.1 Classification of LRs: qualitative and (semi-)quantitative

LR value	Qualitative classification: Change in probability of disease [14]	Approximate change in probability (%) [32]
≤0.1	Very large decrease	–
0.1	Large decrease	–45
≤0.2	Large decrease	–30
0.3	Moderate decrease	–25
0.4	Moderate decrease	–20
≤0.5	Moderate decrease	–15
0.5 < NLR ≤ 1.0	Slight decrease	–
1.0		0
1.0 < PLR < 2.0	Slight increase	–
2.0	Moderate increase	+15
3.0	Moderate increase	+20
4.0	Moderate increase	+25
≤5.0	Moderate increase	+30
6.0	Large increase	+35
8.0	Large increase	+40
≤10.0	Large increase	+45
≥ 10.0	Very large increase	–

Worked Example: Result-Specific LR

The "attended with" (AW) sign has been proposed as a useful screening test for the diagnosis of cognitive impairment. In a screening test accuracy study in a large consecutive patient cohort (N = 1209), AW sign was observed in 473 of 507 patients with a final clinical diagnosis of major or minor neurocognitive disorder (by DSM-5 criteria) and in 306 of 702 patients with no cognitive impairment [21].

Hence, the probability of AW given cognitive impairment is 473/507 = 0.933, and the probability of AW given no cognitive impairment is 306/702 = 0.436. Note that these values are equivalent to the true positive rate (TPR) or sensitivity of the test and the false positive rate (FPR). Hence the result-specific likelihood ratio is given by:

$$LR = p(R_i|\,D+)/p(R_i|\,D-)$$
$$= TPR/FPR$$
$$= 0.933/0.436$$
$$= 2.14$$

Following the qualitative classification of likelihood ratios described by Jaeschke et al. [14], LR = 2.14 represents a moderate increase in the probability of disease.

Worked Examples: Category-Specific PLR, NLR

In a screening test accuracy study of the MACE [17], at the MACE cut-off $\leq$ 20/30, Sens = 0.912 and Spec = 0.707 for dementia diagnosis (Sect. 2.2.1).

Hence, the positive likelihood ratio (PLR) at this cut-off is:

$$PLR = Sens/(1 - Spec)$$
$$= 0.912/(1 - 0.707)$$
$$= 3.11$$

Following the qualitative classification of likelihood ratios described by Jaeschke et al. [14], PLR = 3.11 represents a moderate increase in the probability of disease.

The negative likelihood ratio (NLR) at this cut-off is:

$$NLR = (1 - Sens)/Spec$$
$$= (1 - 0.912)/0.707$$
$$= 0.124$$

Following the qualitative classification of likelihood ratios described by Jaeschke et al. [14], NLR = 0.124 represents a large decrease in the probability of disease.

Note that these results could also be obtained from the raw study data (see Fig. 2.2). For PLR, the probability of MACE $\leq$20/30 given dementia is 104/114 = 0.912 (equivalent to sensitivity or true positive rate) and the probability of MACE $\leq$ 20/30 given no dementia is 188/641 = 0.293 (equivalent to false positive rate; Sect. 2.2.2). Hence the category-specific positive likelihood ratio is given by:

$$PLR = p(T + | D+)/p(T + | D-)$$
$$= TPR/FPR$$
$$= 0.912/0.293$$
$$= 3.11$$

For NLR, the probability of MACE > 20/30 given dementia is $10/114 = 0.088$ (equivalent to false negative rate; Sect. 2.2.2) and the probability of MACE >20/30 given no dementia is $453/641 = 0.707$ (equivalent to specificity or true negative rate). Hence the category-specific negative likelihood ratio is given by:

$$NLR = p(T- \mid D+)/p(T- \mid D-)$$
$$= FNR/TNR$$
$$= 0.088/0.707$$
$$= 0.124$$

Confidence (or compatibility) intervals (CI; Sect. 1.7) may be easily calculated for LR values by applying the log method to data from the four cells of the 2×2 contingency table [15].

$$\log_e(LR) + /-[1.96 \times SE(\log_e LR)]$$

where, using algebraic notation:

$$SE(\log_e LR) = \sqrt{[1/a - 1/(a+c) + 1/b - 1/(b+d)]}$$

Worked Examples: Confidence Intervals For LRs

In a screening test accuracy study of MACE [17], at the MACE cut-off of $\leq$ 20/30 the outcomes using algebraic notation (Fig. 1.2) were a = 104, b = 188, c = 10, d = 453. As previously shown, PLR = 3.11 and NLR = 0.124.

Hence the 95% confidence intervals (95% CI) for PLR and NLR are:

$$95\%CI = [1.96 \times SE(\log_e LR)]$$
$$SE(\log_e LR) = \sqrt{[1/a - 1/(a+c) + 1/b - 1/(b+d)]}$$
$$= \sqrt{[1/104 - 1/(114) + 1/188 - 1/(641)]}$$
$$= 0.0678$$
$$95\%CI = 1.96 \times 0.0678 = 0.133$$
$$PLR = 3.11(95\%CI = 2.72 - 3.55)$$
$$NLR = 0.124(95\%CI = 0.109 - 0.142)$$

As LRs are derived from sensitivity and specificity, like these measures they are algebraically unrelated to the base rate, P. However, as is the case for Sens and Spec, in practice LRs are not independent of prevalence [3].

LRs vary with test cut-off [17] (see also Fig. 8.9) and hence with Q. Quality likelihood ratios, QPLR and QNLR, may be calculated (Sect. 6.3.4).

Rather than dichotomising outcomes with a single cut-off, dividing continuous data into intervals and calculating interval likelihood ratios (ILRs) is possible [5] (Sect. 8.5.2).

Calculation of LRs also provides a method for combining the results of multiple tests, assuming conditional independence of the tests in the presence and absence of the target diagnosis:

$$Post - test\,odds = Pre - test\,odds \times LR_1 \times LR_2 + \ldots LR_n$$

Combination of test results using this method is further considered in Sect. 8.2.1.

2.3.6 Post-test Odds; Net Harm to Net Benefit (H/B) Ratio

Post-test odds may be calculated as the product of PLR and the pre-test odds (Sect. 1.3.3), a form of Bayesian updating:

$$Post - test\,odds = Pre - test\,odds \times PLR$$
$$= (P/P') \times PLR$$

In probability notation:

$$Post - test\,odds = p(D+)/p(D-) \times PLR$$

Worked Examples: Post-test Odds, Post-test Probability

In the screening test accuracy study of MACE [17], the pre-test odds of dementia were 0.178 (Sect. 1.3.3). The positive likelihood ratio, PLR, of MACE using the cut-off $\leq 20/30$ was 3.11 (Sect. 2.3.5).

Hence the post-test odds of dementia using MACE cut-off $\leq 20/30$ are:

$$Post - test\,odds = Pre - test\,odds \times PLR$$
$$= 0.178 \times 3.11$$
$$= 0.553$$

If desired, post-test odds may be converted back to a post-test probability, for comparison with the pre-test probability:

$$Post - test\,probability = Post - test\,odds/(1 + post - test\,odds)$$

$$= 0.553/1.553$$
$$= 0.356$$

This may be compared with the pre-test probability ($=$ prevalence) in this cohort of 0.151 (Sect. 1.3.2), indicating the added value of the test.

McGee [32] advocated some simple (semi-)quantitative rules to obviate these calculations between pre- and post-test odds and probabilities, such that PLR values of 2, 5, and 10 increased the probability by 15%, 30%, and 45% respectively, whereas NLR values of 0.5, 0.2, and 0.1 decreased the probability by 15%, 30% and 45% respectively (Table 2.1, right hand column). These approximate figures derive from the almost linear relationship of probability and the natural logarithm of odds over the range 10–90%, such that the change in probability may be calculated independent of pre-test probability:

$$\text{Change in probability} = 0.19 \times \log_e(LR)$$

(A similar method may be used to classify values of the Efficiency index semi-quantitatively; see Sect. 5.11).

The post-test odds may also be characterised as the ratio of net harm to net benefit (H/B), that is the harm (H) of treating a person without disease (i.e. a false positive) to the net benefit (B) of treating a person with disease (i.e. a true positive), the latter term equating to the harm of a false negative result [8]. H/B ratio may also be calculated using Bayes' equation:

$$\text{Net Harm}(H)/\text{Net Benefit}(B) = \text{Pre} - \text{test odds} \times \text{PLR}$$
$$= (P/P') \times \text{PLR}$$
$$= (P/P') \times (\text{TPR}/\text{FPR})$$

For the net harm to net benefit (H/B) ratio, higher values are desirable if the harm of a false negative (missing a case) is deemed more significant than the harm of diagnosing a false positive (identifying a non-case as a case), a view most clinicians would hold to (see Sect. 3.2.4 for discussion). A higher H/B ratio means that the test is less likely to miss cases, and hence less likely to incur the harms of false negatives. (This scoring of H/B ratio may seem counterintuitive if one thinks solely of "harms" and "benefits", hence the important qualification of "net"). Tests with high sensitivity may nevertheless have an undesirably low H/B ratio if they also have poor specificity [23].

This equation is also pertinent to considerations of misclassification cost (Sect. 3.2.4) as harms are sometimes characterised as "costs" and hence the term cost:benefit ratio is sometimes used. Also, since TPR/FPR is equivalent to the slope of the receiver operating characteristic (ROC) curve ([13], p.68, 157, 171), this is also relevant to the setting of test cut-offs using the ROC curve (Sect. 7.3).

2.3.7   Conditional Probability Plot

A conditional probability plot may be used to illustrate graphically the variation in post-test probability across the complete range of pre-test probabilities (Fig. 2.3). Two curves are generated: one for $p(D+ | T+)$, or PPV; and one for $p(D+ | T-)$, or FRR (Table 2.2, central columns, MACE cut-off $\leq$ 20/30). The point at P = 0.5 on the test-positive plot corresponds to the standardized positive predictive value (SPPV; Sect. 2.3.3) and at P = 0.5 on the test-negative plot corresponds to (1 – SNPV). The diagonal line corresponds to the situation where a test has LR = 1, such that pre-test and post-test probabilities are equal and the test result contributes no information.

Clearly, the shape of the conditional probability plot is dependent on the chosen test cut-off (i.e. Q). For example, contrast the plots for MACE cut-off $\leq$ 20/30 (Fig. 2.3) with MACE cut-offs $\leq$ 25/30 (from the index study [11]; Fig. 2.4 and Table 2.2, right hand columns) and $\leq$15/30 (Fig. 2.5 and Table 2.2, left hand columns), in other words a high Sens low Spec (or "liberal") cut-off versus a low Sens high Spec (or "conservative") cut-off.

With the higher cut-off ($\leq$ 25/30; Fig. 2.4), the test-negative plot is further from the LR = 1 diagonal than with the lower cut-off ($\leq$ 15/30; Fig. 2.5), indicating that $p(D+ | T-)$ is extremely low at this test threshold, suggesting this it is very good for ruling out disease (few false negatives, high NPV).

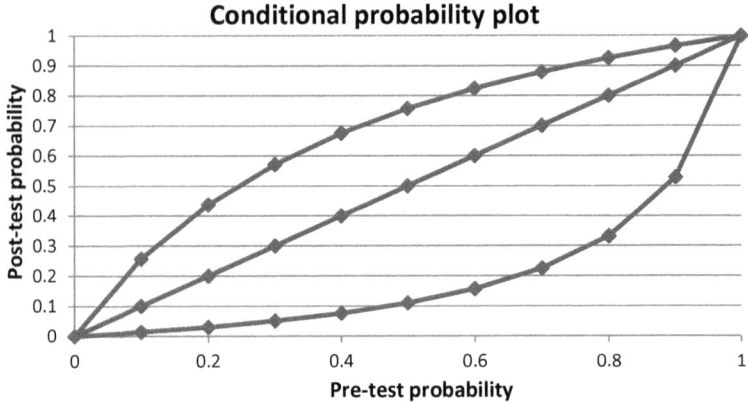

Fig. 2.3 Conditional probability plot of post-test probability (dependent variable; y axis) vs pre-test probability (independent variable; x axis) of MACE for dementia diagnosis at cut-off $\leq$ 20/30 (data from [22], p.157). Upper curve (test positive) corresponds to PPV (see Fig. 3.10); lower curve (test negative) corresponds to FRR (see Fig. 3.11)

Table 2.2 Values of PPV and FRR for dementia diagnosis at fixed MACE cut-offs of $\leq 15/30$, $\leq 20/30$, and $\leq 25/30$ at various prevalence levels, correspondingly to Figs. 2.5, 2.3 and 2.4 respectively

P, P′	MACE cut-off $\leq 15/30$		MACE cut-off $\leq 20/30$		MACE cut-off $\leq 25/30$	
	PPV	FRR	PPV	FRR	PPV	FRR
0.1, 0.9	0.411	0.041	0.257	0.014	0.138	0.003
0.2, 0.8	0.610	0.087	0.437	0.030	0.266	0.007
0.3, 0.7	0.729	0.141	0.571	0.051	0.383	0.012
0.4, 0.6	0.810	0.203	0.675	0.076	0.491	0.019
0.5, 0.5	0.862	0.276	0.757	0.110	0.591	0.028
0.6, 0.4	0.904	0.364	0.824	0.157	0.685	0.041
0.7, 0.3	0.936	0.471	0.879	0.225	0.771	0.063
0.8, 0.2	0.962	0.605	0.926	0.332	0.853	0.103
0.9, 0.1	0.983	0.775	0.966	0.528	0.929	0.205

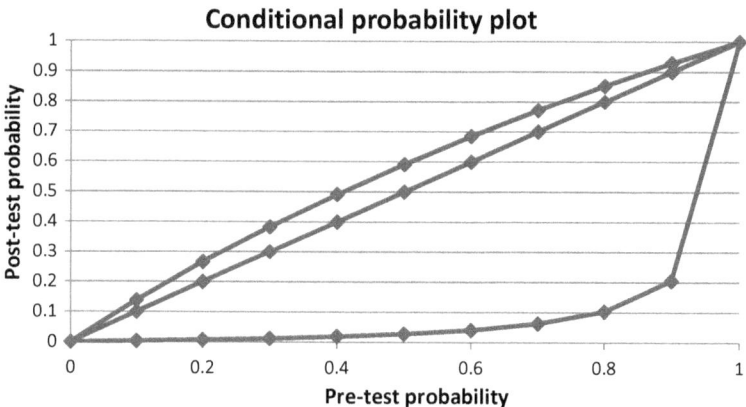

Fig. 2.4 Conditional probability plot of post-test probability vs pre-test probability of MACE for dementia diagnosis at cut-off $\leq 25/30$ (i.e. high Sens, low Spec, "liberal" cut-off). Compare with Figs. 2.3 and 2.5

The test-positive line is closer to $LR = 1$ for the higher cut-off ($\leq 25/30$), indicating that $p(D+ \mid T+)$ at this threshold is not as effective as the lower threshold ($\leq 15/30$) for ruling disease in (lower PLR).

Dependence of test parameters on Q is considered further in the next chapter, but suffice it to say here that these conditional probability plots at different test cut-offs effectively illustrate the heuristic "SnNOut" and "SpPIn" rules (Sect. 3.2.3) [25].

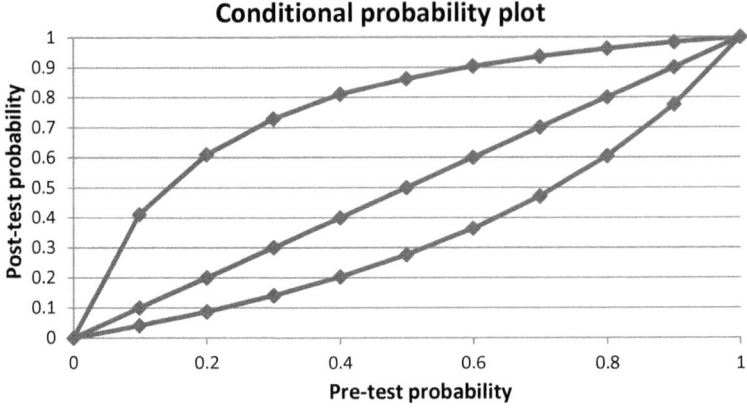

Fig. 2.5 Conditional probability plot of post-test probability vs pre-test probability of MACE for dementia diagnosis at cut-off ≤15/30 (i.e. low Sens, high Spec, "conservative" cut-off). Compare with Figs. 2.3 and 2.4

2.3.8 Positive and Negative Predictive Ratios (PPR, NPR)

Linn described two measures which are analogous to likelihood ratios (Sect. 2.3.5) but based on predictive values (Sect. 2.3.1), rather than Sens and Spec (Sect. 2.2.1), and named "predictive ratios" [30].

The positive predictive ratio (PPR) is given by:

$$PPR = PPV/(1 - NPV)$$
$$= PPV/FRR$$

In literal notation:

$$PPR = [TP/(TP + FP)]/[FN/(FN + TN)]$$
$$= [TP/q]/[FN/q']$$
$$= [TP \cdot q']/[FN \cdot q]$$

In algebraic notation:

$$PPR = [a/(a + b)]/[c/(c + d)]$$
$$= [a \cdot (c + d)]/[c \cdot (a + b)]$$
$$= [a \cdot q']/[c \cdot q]$$

In probability notation:

$$PPR = p(D + | T+)/p(D + | T-)$$

By Bayes' equation:

$$PPR = [p(T+|D+) \cdot p(D+)/p(T+|D+) \cdot p(D+) + p(T+|D-) \cdot p(D-)]$$
$$\div [p(T-|D+) \cdot p(D+)/p(T-|D+) \cdot p(D+) + p(T-|D-) \cdot p(D-)]$$

The negative predictive ratio (NPR) is given by:

$$NPR = (1 - PPV)/NPV$$
$$= FDR/NPV$$

In literal notation:

$$NPR = [FP/(TP + FP)]/[TN/(FN + TN)]$$
$$= [FP/q]/[TN/q']$$
$$= [FP \cdot q']/[TN \cdot q]$$

In algebraic notation:

$$NPR = [b/(a + b)]/[d/(c + d)]$$
$$= [b \cdot (c + d)]/[d \cdot (a + b)]$$
$$= [b \cdot q']/[d \cdot q]$$

In probability notation:

$$NPR = p(D - | T+)/p(D - | T-)$$

By Bayes' equation:

$$NPR = [p(T+|D-) \cdot p(D-)/p(T+|D-) \cdot p(D-) + p(T+|D+) \cdot p(D+)]$$
$$\div p(T-|D-) \cdot p(D-)/p(T-|D-) \cdot p(D-) + p(T-|D+) \cdot p(D+)$$

Worked Examples: PPR, NPR

In a screening test accuracy study of the MACE [17], at the MACE cut-off $\leq 20/30$, PPV = 0.356 and NPV = 0.978 (Sect. 2.3.1).

Hence, the positive predictive ratio (PPR) at this cut-off is:

$$PPR = PPV/(1 - NPV)$$
$$= 0.356/(1 - 0.978)$$
$$= 0.356/0.02159$$
$$= 16.49$$

The negative predictive ratio (NPR) is:

$$NPR = (1 - PPV)/NPV$$
$$= (1 - 0.356)/0.978$$
$$= 0.658$$

As for LRs, these results can also be obtained from the raw study data (see Fig. 2.2). For PPR, the probability of dementia given MACE $\leq$20/30 is 104/292 = 0.356 (equivalent to positive predictive value) and the probability of dementia given MACE >20/30 is 10/463 = 0.022 (equivalent to false reassurance rate; Sect. 2.3.2). Hence PPR is given by:

$$PPR = p(D+ \mid T+)/p(D+ \mid T-)$$
$$= PPV/FRR$$
$$= 0.356/0.02159$$
$$= 16.49$$

For NPR, the probability of no dementia given MACE $\leq$ 20/30 is 188/292 = 0.644 (equivalent to false discovery rate; Sect. 2.3.2) and the probability of no dementia given MACE >20/30 is 453/463 = 0.978 (equivalent to negative predictive value). Hence NPR is given by:

$$NPR = p(D- \mid T+)/p(D- \mid T-)$$
$$= FDR/NPV$$
$$= 0.644/0.978$$
$$= 0.658$$

PPR and NPR values are seldom examined in practice [2]. Quality predictive ratios, QPPR and QNPR, may be calculated (Sect. 6.3.5).

2.4   Association-Based Measures

2.4.1   Diagnostic Odds Ratio (DOR) and Error Odds Ratios (EOR)

The diagnostic odds ratio (DOR) or the cross product ratio [6, 7] is the ratio of the product of true positives and true negatives and of false negatives and false positives.
In literal notation:

$$DOR = (TP \times TN)/(FP \times FN)$$

In algebraic notation:

$$DOR = (ad)/(bc)$$

DOR may also be expressed in terms of other previously encountered parameters (Sens, Spec, likelihood ratios, predictive values, and predictive ratios):

$$
\begin{aligned}
DOR &= (Sens \times Spec)/[(1 - Sens) \times (1 - Spec)] \\
&= (Sens \times Spec)/(FNR \times FPR) \\
&= (TPR \times TNR)/(FNR \times FPR) \\
&= [TPR/(1 - TPR)] \times [(1 - FPR)/FPR] \\
&= PLR/NLR \\
&= PPV \times NPV/(1 - PPV) \times (1 - NPV) \\
&= PPV \times NPV/FDR \times FRR \\
&= PPR/NPR
\end{aligned}
$$

Hence, from LRs, in error notation:

$$
\begin{aligned}
DOR &= [(1 - \beta)/\alpha]/[\beta/(1 - \alpha)] \\
&= (1 - \beta)(1 - \alpha)/(\alpha\beta)
\end{aligned}
$$

DOR may range from 0 (if cells a and/or d are zero) to ∞ (if cells b and/or c are zero), with DOR $= 1$ denoting a random classifier (useless test). A qualitative classification of DOR values was suggested by Rosenthal, as: small ~1.5, medium ~2.5, large ~4, and very large ~10 or greater [39].
A rescaling to a weighted kappa statistic with endpoints of 0 (random classifier) and 1 (perfect classifier) has been described [42].

Worked Examples: DOR

In a screening test accuracy study of MACE [17], at the MACE cut-off of $\leq$ 20/30 (Fig. 2.2), TP = 104, FN = 10, FP = 188, and TN = 453.

Hence the value for DOR at this cut-off is:

$$DOR = (TP \times TN)/(FP \times FN)$$
$$= 104 \times 453/188 \times 10$$
$$= 25.06$$

Knowing Sens (0.912) and Spec (0.707) at this cut-off (Sect. 2.2.1), DOR could also be calculated thus:

$$DOR = (Sens \times Spec)/[(1 - Sens) \times (1 - Spec)]$$
$$= 0.912 \times 0.707/(1 - 0.912) \times (1 - 0.707)$$
$$= 0.645/0.088 \times 0.293$$
$$= 25.01$$

Knowing PLR (3.11) and NLR (0.124) at this cut-off (Sect. 2.3.5), DOR could also be calculated thus:

$$DOR = PLR/NLR$$
$$= 3.11/0.124$$
$$= 25.08$$

Knowing PPR (16.49) and NPR (0.658) at this cut-off (Sect. 2.3.8), DOR could also be calculated thus:

$$DOR = PPR/NPR$$
$$= 16.49/0.658$$
$$= 25.06$$

[The slight differences in results relate to rounding errors.]

Following the qualitative classification of DORs described by Rosenthal [39], DOR > 25 represents a very large value.

Confidence (compatibility) intervals (CI) may be easily calculated for DOR values by applying the log method, as for likelihood ratios (Sect. 2.3.5).

DOR has known shortcomings [16, 19]. It treats FN and FP as equally undesirable, which is often not the case in clinical practice (see Sect. 3.2.4). By choosing the best quality of a test and ignoring its weaknesses, it gives the most optimistic results, particularly in populations with very high or very low risk. Ratios become unstable and inflated as the denominator approaches zero, and may be zero or infinite if one of the classes is nil.

As small differences in one cell value can drastically alter DOR, use of the logarithm of the DOR is sometimes used to compensate. As DOR is a combination of products and quotients this is easily done (either common or natural logs may be used):

$$\log(DOR) = \log(TP) + \log(TN) - \log(FP) - \log(FN)$$
$$= \log(a) + \log(d) - \log(b) - \log(c)$$

Log (DOR) may also be calculated from Sens and Spec, specifically from their logits (logarithms of odds):

$$DOR = (Sens \times Spec)/[(1 - Sens) \times (1 - Spec)]$$
$$\log(DOR) = \log[Sens/(1 - Sens)] + \log[Spec/(1 - Spec)]$$
$$= logit(Sens) + logit(Spec)$$

Worked Example: Log(DOR)

In a screening test accuracy study of MACE [17], at the MACE cut-off of $\leq 20/30$, Sens $= 0.912$ and Spec $= 0.707$ (Sect. 2.2.1).

Hence the value for log (DOR) at this cut-off, using common logs, is:

$$\log(DOR) = \log[Sens/(1 - Sens)] + \log[Spec/(1 - Spec)]$$
$$= \log[0.912/0.088] + \log[0.707/0.293]$$
$$= 1.0155 + 0.38255$$
$$= 1.3981$$
$$Antilog = DOR = 25.01$$

Log_e (DOR) is used as an accuracy parameter in meta-analysis when model fitting summary ROC curves.

The relation of DOR to Sens and Spec may also be seen graphically in the receiver operating characteristic (ROC) plot (Sect. 7.2), and of log (DOR) to log likelihood ratios in the ROC plot in likelihood ratio coordinates (Sect. 7.4.1).

As DOR is related to cut-off and hence Q, a rescaled quality DOR, QDOR, may also be calculated [18] (Sect. 6.4.1).

An error odds ratio (EOR) may also be defined, as the ratio of the product of true positives and false positives and of true negatives and false negatives.

In literal notation:

$$EOR = (TP \times FP)/(FN \times TN)$$

In algebraic notation:

$$EOR = (ab)/(cd)$$

EOR is seldom examined and not recommended [2].

Worked Example: EOR

In a screening test accuracy study of MACE [17], at the MACE cut-off of $\leq$ 20/30 (Fig. 2.2), TP = 104, FN = 10, FP = 188, and TN = 453.
Hence the values for EOR at this cut-off is:

$$EOR = (TP \times FP)/(FN \times TN)$$
$$= 104 \times 188/10 \times 453$$
$$= 4.32$$

2.4.2 Positive and Negative Clinical Utility Indexes (PCUI, NCUI)

The clinical utility indexes developed by Mitchell [34] calculate the value of a diagnostic method for ruling in or ruling out a diagnosis.
Positive clinical utility index (PCUI; also sometimes denoted CUI+) is given by:

$$PCUI = Sens \times PPV$$
$$= TPR \times PPV$$

In literal notation:

$$PCUI = TP/(TP + FN) \times TP/(TP + FP)$$
$$= TP^2/[(TP + FN) \cdot (TP + FP)]$$
$$= TP^2/[p \cdot q]$$

In algebraic notation:

$$PCUI = a/(a + c) \times a/(a + b)$$
$$= a^2/[(a + c) \cdot (a + b)]$$
$$= a^2/[p \cdot q]$$

This parameter has also been termed the Screening Marker Index [36].
Negative clinical utility index (NCUI; also sometimes denoted CUI−) is given by:

$$NCUI = Spec \times NPV$$
$$= TNR \times NPV$$

In literal notation:

$$NCUI = TN/(FP + TN) \times TN/(FN + TN)$$
$$= TN^2/[(FP + TN) \cdot (FN + TN)]$$
$$= TN^2/[p' \cdot q']$$

In algebraic notation:

$$NCUI = d/(b + d) \times d/(c + d)$$
$$= d^2/[(b + d).(c + d)]$$
$$= d^2/[p' \cdot q']$$

Clinical utility index values range from 0 to 1, with higher values better. In addition to the absolute score, the qualitative performance of CUI values may be classified as: excellent ≥ 0.81, good ≥ 0.64, adequate ≥ 0.49, poor ≥ 0.36, or very poor < 0.36 [34].

Worked Examples: PCUI, NCUI

In a screening test accuracy study of the MACE [17], at the MACE cut-off of $\leq 20/30$, Sens $= 0.912$ and Spec $= 0.707$ (Sect. 2.2.1), and PPV $= 0.356$ and NPV $= 0.978$ (Sect. 2.3.1).

Hence, the positive clinical utility index (PCUI) at this cut-off is:

$$PCUI = Sens \times PPV$$
$$= 0.912 \times 0.356$$
$$= 0.325$$

Following the qualitative classification of clinical utility indexes described by Mitchell [32], PCUI $= 0.325$ is very poor.

The negative clinical utility index (NCUI) is:

$$NCUI = Spec \times NPV$$
$$= 0.707 \times 0.978$$
$$= 0.691$$

Following the qualitative classification of clinical utility indexes described by Mitchell [32], NCUI $= 0.691$ is good.

Rescaled, quality CUIs [18], QPCUI and QNCUI, may also be calculated (Sect. 6.4.2).

2.4.3 Positive and Negative Clinical Disutility Indexes (PCDI, PCDI)

Clinical disutility indexes (CDI) may also be developed (first described in [24], p.44–5), to calculate the limitation of a diagnostic method for ruling in or ruling out a diagnosis.

Positive clinical disutility index (PCDI; also sometimes denoted CDI $+$) is given by:

$$PCDI = (1 - Sens) \times (1 - PPV)$$
$$= FNR \times FDR$$

This is a measure of incorrectly ruling out.

Negative clinical disutility index (NCDI; also sometimes denoted CDI-) is given by:

$$NCDI = (1 - Spec) \times (1 - NPV)$$
$$= FPR \times FRR$$

This is a measure of incorrectly ruling in.

As for CUI, clinical disutility index values range from 0 to 1, but with lower values better. In addition to the absolute score, the qualitative performance of CDI might be classified, after CUI, as: very poor $\geq$ 0.81, poor $\geq$ 0.64, adequate $\geq$ 0.49, good $\geq$ 0.36, or excellent < 0.36 ([24], p.44–5).

Worked Examples: PCDI, PCDI

In a screening test accuracy study of the MACE [17], at the MACE cut-off of $\leq$20/30, Sens = 0.912 and Spec = 0.707 (Sect. 2.2.1), and PPV = 0.356 and NPV = 0.978 (Sect. 2.3.1). Hence FNR = 0.088 and FPR = 0.293 (Sect. 2.2.2) and FDR = 0.644 and FRR = 0.022 (Sect. 2.3.2).

Hence, the positive clinical disutility index (PCDI) at this cut-off is:

$$PCDI = FNR \times FDR$$
$$= 0.088 \times 0.644$$
$$= 0.057$$

Following the suggested qualitative classification of clinical disutility indexes, PCDI = 0.057 is excellent, suggesting the test is unlikely to rule out the diagnosis incorrectly.

The negative clinical disutility index (NCDI) is:

$$NCDI = FPR \times FRR$$
$$= 0.293 \times 0.022$$
$$= 0.006$$

Following the suggested qualitative classification of clinical disutility indexes, NCDI = 0.006 is excellent, suggesting the test is unlikely to rule in the diagnosis incorrectly.

Rescaled, quality CDIs, QPCDI and QNCDI, may also be calculated (Sect. 6.4.3).

References

1. Altman DG, Bland JM. Diagnostic tests 2: Predictive values. BMJ. 1994;309:102.
2. Bossuyt PMM. Clinical validity: defining biomarker performance. Scand J Clin Lab Invest. 2010;70(Suppl242):46–52.
3. Brenner H, Gefeller O. Variation of sensitivity, specificity, likelihood ratios and predictive values with disease prevalence. Stat Med. 1997;16:981–91.
4. Brismar J, Jacobsson B. Definition of terms used to judge the efficacy of diagnostic tests: a graphic approach. AJR Am J Roentgenol. 1990;155:621–3.
5. Brown MD, Reeves MJ. Interval likelihood ratios: another advantage for the evidence-based diagnostician. Ann Emerg Med. 2003;42:292–7.
6. Edwards AWF. The measure of association in a 2×2 table. J R Stat Soc Ser A. 1963;126:109–14.
7. Glas AS, Lijmer JG, Prins MH, Bonsel GJ, Bossuyt PM. The diagnostic odds ratio: a single indicator of test performance. J Clin Epidemiol. 2003;56:1129–35.
8. Habibzadeh F, Habibzadeh P, Yadollahie M. On determining the most appropriate test cut-off value: the case of tests with continuous results. Biochem Med (Zagreb). 2016;26:297–307.
9. Heston TF. Standardizing predictive values in diagnostic imaging research. J Magn Reson Imaging. 2011;33:505.
10. Heston TF. Standardized predictive values. J Magn Reson Imaging. 2014;39:1338.
11. Hlatky MA, Mark DB, Harrell FE Jr, Lee KL, Califf RM, Pryor DB. Rethinking sensitivity and specificity. Am J Cardiol. 1987;59:1195–8.
12. Hsieh S, McGrory S, Leslie F, Dawson K, Ahmed S, Butler CR, et al. The Mini-Addenbrooke's Cognitive Examination: a new assessment tool for dementia. Dement Geriatr Cogn Disord. 2015;39:1–11.
13. Hunink MGM, Weinstein MC, Wittenberg E, Drummond MF, Pliskin JS, Wong JB, et al. Decision making in health and medicine. Integrating evidence and values. 2nd edn. Cambridge: Cambridge University Press; 2014.
14. Jaeschke R, Guyatt G, Sackett DL. User's guide to the medical literature. III. How to use an article about a diagnostic test. B. What are the results and will they help me in caring for my patients? JAMA. 1994;271:703–7.

15. Katz D, Baptista J, Azen SP, Pike MC. Obtaining confidence intervals for the risk ratio in cohort studies. Biometrics. 1978;34:469–74.
16. Kraemer HC. Evaluating medical tests. Objective and quantitative guidelines. Newbery Park, California: Sage; 1992.
17. Larner AJ. MACE for diagnosis of dementia and MCI: examining cut-offs and predictive values. Diagnostics (Basel). 2019;9:E51.
18. Larner AJ. Applying Kraemer's Q (positive sign rate): some implications for diagnostic test accuracy study results. Dement Geriatr Cogn Dis Extra. 2019;9:389–96.
19. Larner AJ. New unitary metrics for dementia test accuracy studies. Prog Neurol Psychiatry. 2019;23(3):21–5.
20. Larner AJ. Mini-Addenbrooke's Cognitive Examination (MACE): a useful cognitive screening instrument in older people? Can Geriatr J. 2020;23:199–204.
21. Larner AJ. The "attended alone" and "attended with" signs in the assessment of cognitive impairment: a revalidation. Postgrad Med. 2020;132:595–600.
22. Larner AJ. Manual of screeners for dementia. Pragmatic test accuracy studies. London: Springer; 2020.
23. Larner AJ. Cognitive screening instruments for dementia: comparing metrics of test limitation. Dement Neuropsychol. 2021;15:458–63.
24. Larner AJ. The 2 × 2 matrix. Contingency, confusion and the metrics of binary classification. London: Springer; 2021.
25. Larner AJ. Re: diagnostic reasoning: conditional probability plots illustrate "SnNOut" and SpPIn" rules. https://www.bmj.com/content/376/bmj-2021-064389/rr-0. (08 Feb 2022)
26. Larner AJ. Cognitive screening in older people using Free-Cog and Mini-Addenbrooke's Cognitive Examination (MACE). Preprints.org. 2023;2023:2023040237. https://doi.org/10.20944/preprints202304.0237.v1
27. Larrabee GJ, Barry DTR. Diagnostic classification statistics and diagnostic validity of malingering assessment. In: Larrabee GJ, editor. Assessment of malingered neuropsychological deficits. Oxford: Oxford University Press; 2007. p. 14–26.
28. Leeflang MM, Bossuyt PM, Irwig L. Diagnostic test accuracy may vary with prevalence: implications for evidence-based diagnosis. J Clin Epidemiol. 2009;62:5–12.
29. Leeflang MM, Rutjes AW, Reitsma JB, Hooft L, Bossuyt PM. Variation of a test's sensitivity and specificity with disease prevalence. CMAJ. 2013;185:E537–44.
30. Linn S. New patient-oriented diagnostic test characteristics analogous to the likelihood ratios conveyed information on trustworthiness. J Clin Epidemiol. 2005;58:450–7.
31. Mathuranath PS, Nestor PJ, Berrios GE, Rakowicz W, Hodges JR. A brief cognitive test battery to differentiate Alzheimer's disease and frontotemporal dementia. Neurology. 2000;55:1613–20.
32. McGee S. Simplifying likelihood ratios. J Gen Intern Med. 2002;17:647–50.
33. Mioshi E, Dawson K, Mitchell J, Arnold R, Hodges JR. The Addenbrooke's Cognitive Examination Revised: a brief cognitive test battery for dementia screening. Int J Geriatr Psychiatry. 2006;21:1078–85.
34. Mitchell AJ. Sensitivity × PPV is a recognized test called the clinical utility index (CUI+). Eur J Epidemiol. 2011;26:251–2.
35. Neyman J. Outline of statistical treatment of the problem of diagnosis. Public Health Rep. 1947;62:1449–56.
36. Ostergaard SD, Dinesen PT, Foldager L. Quantifying the value of markers in screening programmes. Eur J Epidemiol. 2010;25:151–4.
37. Pauker SG, Kassirer JP. Therapeutic decision making: a cost-benefit analysis. N Engl J Med. 1975;293:229–34.
38. Perera R, Heneghan C. Making sense of diagnostic tests likelihood ratios. Evid Based Med. 2006;11:130–1.
39. Rosenthal JA. Qualitative descriptors of strength of association and effect size. J Soc Serv Res. 1996;21:37–59.

40. Schaefer JT. The critical success index as an indicator of warning skill. Weather Forecast. 1990;5:570–5.
41. Thornbury JR, Fryback DG, Edwards W. Likelihood ratios as a measure of the diagnostic usefulness of excretory urogram information. Radiology. 1975;114:561–5.
42. Warrens MJ. A Kraemer-type rescaling that transforms the odds ratio into the weighted kappa coefficient. Psychometrika. 2010;75:328–30.
43. Yerushalmy J. Statistical problems in assessing methods of medical diagnosis, with special reference to x-ray techniques. Public Health Rep. 1947;62:1432–49.
44. Zimmerman M. Positive predictive value: a clinician's guide to avoid misinterpreting the results of screening tests. J Clin Psychiatry. 2022;83:22com14513.

Chapter 3
Paired Complementary Measures

Contents

3.1 Introduction

This chapter considers complementary paired measures of discrimination. Conditional probability measures may be described as complementary when they necessarily sum to unity. The summation principle that probabilities add to 1 holds for a mutually exclusive and collectively exhaustive set of possibilities.

This formulation has already been encountered when describing the marginal probabilities of the 2×2 matrix, namely P, Q, and R (or Acc), and their complements P', Q', and R' (or Inacc) (Sect. 1.3.2). Another way of conceptualising and describing this relation uses the Boolean "NOT" operator, since P = 1–P', Q = 1–Q', R = 1–R'. Although this logical operation may also be known as negation, this term is not used here since, to my knowledge, there are no arithmetic negations or additive inverse parameters (i.e. necessarily sum to zero) derived from the 2×2 matrix. (Other Boolean operators and their applications to the 2×2 matrix are considered in Sect. 8.2.2).

This chapter reiterates some of the measures previously examined in Chap. 2, as well as looking at other measures, namely accuracy and inaccuracy (Fig. 3.1). As in the previous chapter, the classification of measures as error-based and information-based, following Bossuyt [1], is used. Consideration is also given to correct classification and misclassification rates. The variation of paired measures with pre-test probability or prevalence (P), as described in Sect. 1.3.2, is also illustrated. Variation of measures with Q, the level of test, is also described in passing, with a more detailed treatment deferred to Chap. 6.

		True Status		
		Condition present (= case)	**Condition absent (= non case)**	r'
Test Outcome	**Positive**	True positive [TP] (a)	False positive [FP] (b)	q
	Negative	False negative [FN] (c)	True negative [TN] (d)	q'
		p	p'	r

Paired complementary measures (literal notation only):

Sens (TPR)	=	TP/(TP + FN)	=	TP/p
FNR (1 − Sens)	=	FN/(TP + FN)	=	FN/p
Spec (TNR)	=	TN/(FP + TN)	=	TN/p'
FPR (1 − Spec)	=	FP/(FP + TN)	=	FP/p'
Acc	=	(TP + TN)/(TP + FP + FN + TN)	=	TP +TN/N
Inacc (1 − Acc)	=	FP + FN/(TP + FP + FN + TN)	=	FP + FN/N
PPV	=	TP/(TP + FP)	=	TP/q
FDR (1 − PPV)	=	FP/(TP + FP)	=	FP/q
NPV	=	TN/(FN + TN)	=	TN/q'
FRR (1 − NPV)	=	FN/(FN + TN)	=	FN/q'

Fig. 3.1 2×2 contingency table with literal and algebraic notation, marginal totals, and derived paired complementary measures

3.2 Error-Based Measures

3.2.1 Sensitivity (Sens) and False Negative Rate (FNR)

As previously shown (Sect. 2.2.2), false negative rate (FNR) is the complement of
sensitivity (Sens):

$$FNR = (1 - Sens)$$
$$= (1 - TPR)$$

$$FNR + Sens = 1$$
$$FNR + TPR = 1$$

In error notation, FNR = β, Sens = 1–β (Sect. 1.4).

This is illustrated in the worked examples of Sens (Sect. 2.2.1) and FNR
(Sect. 2.2.2) from a study of the Mini-Addenbrooke's Cognitive Examination
(MACE) [14] showing that the calculated values (Sens = 0.912, FNR = 0.088)
sum to 1. Hence knowing either Sens or FNR will always disclose the other across
the range of test cut-offs (i.e. variation with Q; Fig. 3.2). This also holds for values
rescaled according to Q [12, 15] (Sects. 6.2.1 and 6.2.2).

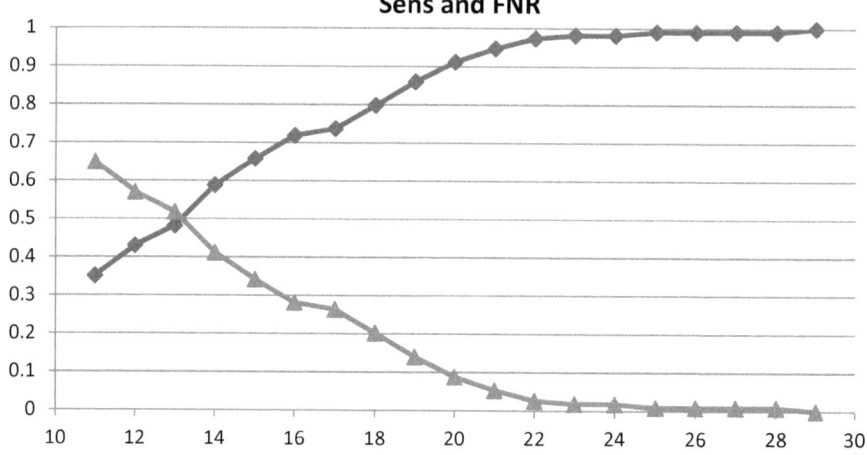

Fig. 3.2 Plot of sensitivity (diamonds) and FNR (triangles) for dementia diagnosis at fixed P (=
0.151) on y axis versus MACE cut-off (x axis) (data from [14])

3.2.2 Specificity (Spec) and False Positive Rate (FPR)

As previously shown (Sect. 2.2.2), false positive rate (FPR) is the complement of specificity (Spec):

$$FPR = (1 - Spec)$$
$$= (1 - TNR)$$

$$FPR + Spec = 1$$
$$FPR + TNR = 1$$

In error notation, FPR = α, Spec = 1–α (Sect. 1.4).

This is illustrated in the worked examples of Spec (Sect. 2.2.1) and FPR (Sect. 2.2.2) from the MACE study [14] showing that the calculated values (Spec = 0.707, FPR = 0.293) sum to 1. Hence knowing either Spec or FPR will always disclose the other across the range of test cut-offs (i.e. variation with Q; Fig. 3.3). This also holds for values rescaled according to Q [12, 15] (Sects. 6.2.1 and 6.2.2).

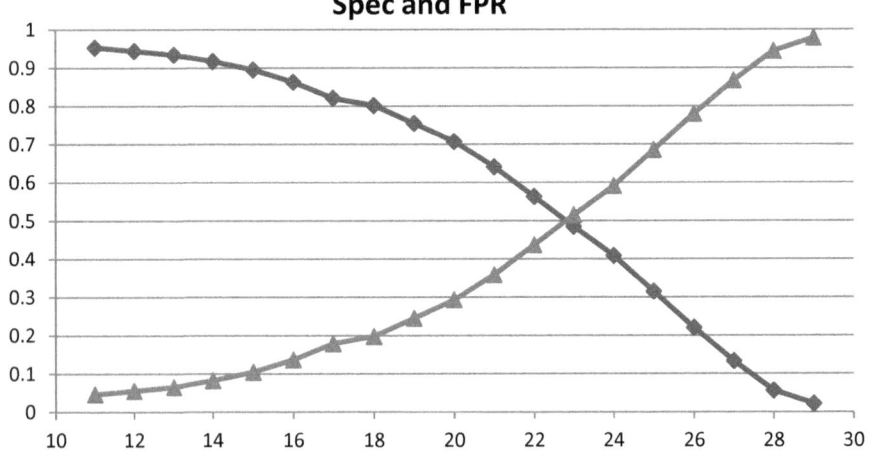

Fig. 3.3 Plot of specificity (diamonds) and FPR (triangles) for dementia diagnosis at fixed P (= 0.151) on y axis versus MACE cut-off (x axis) (data from [14])

3.2.3   "SnNout" and "SpPin" Rules

Gallagher [6] has suggested that the measures of sensitivity and specificity of diagnostic tests ask the wrong question from a clinician's point of view, since they presuppose that a patient either does or does not have a particular disease, in which case the administration of a diagnostic test would not be needed. The clinical utility of sensitivity and specificity is deemed to lie in the mathematical properties of these measures [6].

A very sensitive test will have very few false negatives (FN), but possibly many false positives (FP). Because of the low FNR of a very sensitive test, a negative test result is therefore likely to be a true negative (TN) and hence rules out the diagnosis. This is made explicit in the heuristic "SnNout" rule ([32], p.165–6):

<u>Se</u>nsitive test, <u>N</u>egative result, = diagnosis ruled <u>out</u>

Conversely, a test with low sensitivity has many false negatives, and hence misses cases.

A very specific test will have very few false positives, but possibly many false negatives. Because of the low FPR of a very specific test, a positive test result is therefore likely to be a true positive (TP) and hence rules in the diagnosis. This is made explicit in the heuristic "SpPin" rule ([32], p.165–6):

<u>Sp</u>ecific test, <u>P</u>ositive result, = diagnosis ruled <u>in</u>.

Conversely, a test with low specificity has many false positives, and hence misidentifies non cases as cases.

These heuristics may also be illustrated graphically in conditional probability plots (Sect. 2.3.7; see Figs. 2.3, 2.4, and 2.5) [20]. A knowledge of these heuristics may permit inferences to be made about the value of tests in the absence of empirical data by using clinically reasonable approximations of Sensitivity and Specificity (e.g. [21]).

3.2.4   Classification and Misclassification Rates; Misclassification Costs

The consideration of the complementary paired measures of Sens and FNR (Sect. 3.2.1) and Spec and FPR (Sect. 3.2.2) prompts the inclusion here of a brief discussion of classification and misclassification.

Sens and Spec provide different pieces of information about a test. Is there some way to combine this information into a meaningful outcome parameter? One method has already been encountered, namely likelihood ratios (Sect. 2.3.5), and there are others including Youden index (Sect. 4.2) and receiver operating characteristic (ROC) curves (Sect. 7.2).

However, the simplest way to combine information about Sens and Spec is to sum them, a measure which has been termed "gain in certainty" [4] or overall correct classification rate [30].

$$\text{Correct classification rate} = \text{Sens} + \text{Spec}$$
$$= \text{TPR} + \text{TNR}$$

Of note, unlike most of the parameters considered so far, correct classification rate has a range of 0–2, with higher scores better (technically this is not, therefore, a "rate"). It has been argued that when Sens + Spec = 1 the test provides no information, whilst when the sum is greatest (i.e. = 2) the expected gain is maximised [4].

In literal notation (Fig. 3.1):

$$\text{Correct classification rate} = [\text{TP}/(\text{TP} + \text{FN})] + [\text{TN}/(\text{FP} + \text{TN})]$$
$$= [\text{TP}/\text{p}] + [\text{TN}/\text{p}']$$

In algebraic notation:

$$\text{Correct classification rate} = [a/(a + c)] + [d/(b + d)]$$
$$= [a/\text{p}] + [d/\text{p}']$$

In error notation (see Fig. 1.5):

$$\text{Correct classification rate} = (1-\beta) + (1-\alpha)$$

This summation of Sens and Spec is little used in clinical practice (e.g. [9], p.190; [24], p.100). The Youden index [34] is more frequently used (Sect. 4.2).

The term "misclassification rate" is potentially ambiguous, being sometimes used for the parameter called "proportion incorrect" (Sect. 1.3.2) or "inaccuracy" or "error rate" (Sect. 3.2.5). Here, the usage of Perkins and Schisterman for "misclassification rate" [30] is followed:

$$\text{Misclassification rate} = (1 - \text{Sens}) + (1 - \text{Spec})$$
$$= \text{FNR} + \text{FPR}$$
$$= 2 - (\text{Sens} + \text{Spec})$$

Misclassification rate has a range of 0–2, with lower scores better.
In literal notation (Fig. 3.1):

$$\text{Misclassification rate} = [\text{FN}/(\text{FN} + \text{TP})] + [\text{FP}/(\text{FP} + \text{TN})]$$
$$= [\text{FN}/\text{p}] + [\text{FP}/\text{p}']$$

In algebraic notation:

$$\text{Misclassification rate} = [c/(a+c)]+[b/(b+d)]$$
$$= [c/p] + [b/p']$$

In error notation (see Fig. 1.5):

$$\text{Misclassification rate} = \beta + \alpha$$

Minimisation of the misclassification rate underpins some methods to define optimal cut-offs on receiver operating characteristic (ROC) curves (Sects. 7.3.1 and 7.3.2).

Worked Example: Correct Classification Rate and Misclassification Rate

The Mini-Addenbrooke's Cognitive Examination (MACE) [10] was examined in a screening test accuracy study [14]. At the MACE cut-off of ≤20/30, values for Sens and Spec were 0.912 and 0.707 (Sect. 2.2.1) and hence for FPR and FNR were 0.293 and 0.088 respectively (Sect. 2.2.2).

Hence the value for the correct classification rate at this cut-off was:

$$\text{Correct classification rate} = \text{TPR} + \text{TNR}$$
$$= 0.912 + 0.707$$
$$= 1.619$$

The value for the misclassification rate was:

$$\text{Misclassification rate} = \text{FNR} + \text{FPR}$$
$$= 0.088 + 0.293$$
$$= 0.381$$

Misclassification rates of other cognitive screening instruments have also been reported [19].

Hence correct classification rate and misclassification rate sum to 2:

$$\text{Correct classification rate} + \text{Misclassification rate} = \text{Sens} + \text{Spec} + (1 - \text{Sens})$$
$$+ (1 - \text{Spec}) = 2$$

Their complement (sum to unity) is the Youden index (Y) (see Sect. 4.2 for the derivation of Y):

$$\text{Correct classification rate} = \text{Sens} + \text{Spec}$$
$$Y = \text{Sens} + \text{Spec} - 1$$
$$\text{Correct classification rate} = Y + 1$$
$$\text{Misclassification rate} = \text{FNR} + \text{FPR}$$
$$Y = 1 - (\text{FNR} + \text{FPR})$$
$$\text{Misclassification rate} = 1 - Y$$

Distinction should be drawn between this misclassification rate and another parameter, called misclassification cost. Evidently, both FP and FN classifications have costs (see also the discussion of net harm to net benefit (H/B) ratio in Sect. 2.3.6 [19]). Possible methods to quantify test costs date to Peirce's "utility of the method" in the nineteenth century [29].

In the context of diagnostic or screening test accuracy studies, it may be argued that high test sensitivity in order to identify all true positives, hence with very few false negatives, is more acceptable than tests with low sensitivity but high specificity which risk false negatives (i.e. miss true positives), since the cost of a FN error may be high. Indeed, Youden ([34], p.32) spoke of an "instinctive reaction against a test that is subject to false negatives" since a missed diagnosis may mean missed treatment with resulting disability and even death for a patient. This argument also supposes that the cost of a FP error is not so serious: a healthy patient may be subjected to extra screening and possibly inappropriate treatment unnecessarily. However, the potential ramifications of FP error should not be underestimated, as these may be "profoundly transformational on a personal level" ([25], p.38–9,362,363). Nevertheless, medicine's characteristic (default) decision-rule "that it is better to impute disease than to deny it and risk overlooking or missing it" ([5], p.255) has long been recognised by sociologists of medicine, and the consequences of "nondisease" [26] (i.e. FP resolved to TN) are not necessarily neutral.

Expected benefits (B) and costs (C) at each test cut-off may be expressed as "expected costs" (EC) [12, 31]:

$$\text{EC} = C_{FP} \times \text{FP} + C_{FN} \times \text{FN} - B_{TN} \times \text{TN} - B_{TP} \times \text{TP}$$

The test threshold, c^*, with the lowest EC, is the optimal threshold.
This may also be expressed as a cost ratio (Cr):

$$\text{Cr} = B_{TP} - C_{FN}/B_{TP} + B_{TN} - C_{FN} - C_{FP}$$

The term $(B_{TP} - C_{FN})$ represents the difference in costs if patients with disease (D+) are classified correctly or not, whilst the term $(B_{TN} - C_{FP})$ represents the difference in costs if healthy individuals (D–) are classified correctly or not. Hence Cr is the costs for diseased relative to total costs, or the ratio of relative costs. Cr ranges from 0 to 1. When Cr = 0.5, the difference in costs between correct (T+) and incorrect (T–) test classification is equal for healthy (D–) and diseased (D+) persons. When

Cr = 1, difference in costs is much higher for persons with disease (i.e. FN); when Cr = 0 the difference in costs is much higher for healthy persons (i.e. FP). In most disease screening situations, one anticipates Cr to tend toward 1, since FN errors have higher cost [31].

This notation may also be used in the expression of the net harm to net benefit (H/B) ratio (Sect. 2.3.6). As benefits may be expressed as negative costs if desired [27], and indeed all may be understood as cost expressions [11], then $B_{TP} = C_{TP}$ and $B_{TN} = C_{TN}$. Hence the term $C_{FP} - C_{TN}$ is equal to the net costs of treating a non-diseased patient (harm of FP), and the term $C_{FN} - C_{TP}$ is equal to the net benefits of treating a diseased patient [11] or net costs of not treating a diseased patient (harm of FN):

$$\text{Net Harm(H)}/\text{Net Benefit(B)} = C_{FP} - C_{TN}/C_{FN} - C_{TP}$$

As the misclassification of non-diseased (FN) carries the highest cost, $C_{FN} \gg C_{TP}$, then ideally H/B ratio values should be as high as possible (Sect. 2.3.6) [19].

The ratio of harms of FP to FN (treating a FP unnecessarily to not treating a TP) is also used in methods for determining optimal test cut-off from the receiver operating characteristic (ROC) curve (Sect. 7.3.1) [8].

Another term sometimes used is a relative misclassification cost, defined as FP/TP (literal notation) or b/a (algebraic notation). This is used, for example [28], in a method which gives weighting to the difference in Sens and Spec (ΔSens, ΔSpec) of two tests, hence a weighted comparison (WC), taking into account the relative misclassification cost of false positive diagnosis and also disease prevalence (P), as expressed in the equation:

$$\text{WC} = \Delta\text{Sens} + \left[(1 - P/P) \times (FP/TP) \times \Delta\text{Spec}\right]$$

The relative misclassification cost, FP/TP, seeks to define how many false positives a true positive is worth, a potentially difficult estimate. An arbitrary value of FP/TP = 0.1 may be set [13, 23]. The WC equation does not ostensibly take false negatives into account, but the [(1–P/P) × (FP/TP)] term resembles the net harm to net benefit (H/B) ratio definition (derived in Sect. 2.3.6), where the benefit of TP may be equated to the harm of a FN result.

The question of the relative cost of FP and FN also arises with respect to those measures which assume FN and FP to be equally undesirable, e.g. diagnostic odds ratio (Sect. 2.4.1), Accuracy (Sect. 3.2.5), and Youden index (Sect. 4.2). In all these situations, a trade-off between benefits and costs (sometimes painful) needs to be made.

3.2.5   Accuracy (Acc) and Inaccuracy (Inacc)

Accuracy (Acc) is the sum of true positives and true negatives divided by the total number of patients tested. Acc ranges from 0 to 1, with higher values better.

In literal notation (Fig. 3.1):

$$Acc = (TP + TN)/(TP + FP + FN + TN)$$
$$= (TP + TN)/N$$

In algebraic notation:

$$Acc = a + d/(a + b + c + d)$$
$$= a + d/N$$

and in terms of marginal totals:

$$Acc = r/N$$

This is identical to the value R, defined as one of the marginal probabilities of the basic 2×2 contingency table (Sect. 1.3.2). Acc may also be known correct classification accuracy, effectiveness rate, fraction correct (FC), test efficiency, or posterior probability, or may be stated as the number of individuals correctly classified by the test. Acc, like diagnostic odds ratio (DOR; Sect. 2.4.1), treats FN and FP as equally undesirable, an assumption which is often not the case in clinical practice, and hence a shortcoming of this measure (see Sect. 3.2.4).

It should be noted that "accuracy" is a potentially ambiguous term, as measures of "accuracy" other than Acc are also described [16], including Matthews' correlation coefficient (Sect. 4.5) and the F measure (Sect. 4.8.3), as well as the area under the receiver operating characteristic curve (Sect. 7.2.2).

Acc is calculated using values from both columns of the 2×2 contingency table and hence is sensitive to class imbalance or skews, or in other words it is dependent on disease prevalence, as a weighted average of sensitivity and specificity with weights related to sample prevalence (P and 1–P or P'). Acc may therefore be expressed in terms of P, P', Sens and Spec, such that:

$$Acc = (Sens \cdot P) + (Spec \cdot P')$$

Hence in error notation:

$$Acc = (1-\beta) \cdot P + (1-\alpha) \cdot P'$$

By similar reasoning, Acc is also related to sample cut-off or Q, and to predictive values (Sect. 2.3.1):

$$Acc = (PPV \cdot Q) + (NPV \cdot Q')$$

Worked Example: Acc

In a screening test accuracy study of MACE [14], at the MACE cut-off of $\leq$ 20/30, TP $= 104$, FN $= 10$, FP $= 188$, and TN $= 453$ (see Fig. 2.2).
  Hence the value for Acc at this cut-off is:

$$Acc = (TP + TN)/(TP + FP + FN + TN)$$
$$= (104 + 453)/(104 + 188 + 10 + 453)$$
$$= 0.738$$

Acc may also be expressed in terms of P, P', Sens and Spec. In the MACE study [14], dementia prevalence (P) in the patient cohort (N $= 755$) was 0.151 (Sect. 1.3.2). Values for Sens and Spec at this MACE cut-off are 0.912 and 0.707 respectively (Sect. 2.2.1).
  Hence the value for Acc is:

$$Acc = (Sens \cdot P) + \left(Spec \cdot P'\right)$$
$$= (0.912 \times 0.151) + (0.707 \times 0.849)$$
$$= 0.738$$

Acc may also be expressed in terms of Q, Q', PPV and NPV. In the MACE study [14], Q $= 0.387$ and Q' $= 0.613$ (Sect. 1.3.2). Values for PPV and NPV at this MACE cut-off are 0.356 and 0.978 respectively (Sect. 2.3.1).
  Hence the value for Acc is:

$$Acc = (PPV \cdot Q) + \left(NPV \cdot Q'\right)$$
$$= (0.356 \times 0.387) + (0.978 \times 0.613)$$
$$= 0.738$$

Inaccuracy (Inacc), also sometimes known as error rate, or fraction incorrect, or misclassification rate (although this term has alternate usage; see Sect. 3.2.4), is the complement of Acc:

$$Inacc = (1 - Acc)$$

Hence, Inacc ranges from 0 to 1 with lower values better. Inacc is given by the sum of false positives and false negatives divided by the total number of patients tested.
  In literal notation (Fig. 3.1):

$$Inacc = (FP + FN)/(TP + FP + FN + TN)$$
$$= (FP + FN)/N$$

In algebraic notation:

$$\text{Inacc} = b + c/(a + b + c + d)$$
$$= b + c/N$$

and in terms of marginal totals:

$$\text{Inacc} = r'/N$$

This is identical to the value R', defined as one of the marginal probabilities of the basic 2×2 contingency table (Sect. 1.3.2).

In terms of disease prevalence:

$$\text{Inacc} = (\text{FNR} \cdot P) + (\text{FPR} \cdot P')$$
$$= [(1 - \text{Sens}) \cdot P] + [(1 - \text{Spec}) \cdot P']$$

Hence in error notation:

$$\text{Inacc} = (\beta \cdot P) + (\alpha \cdot P')$$

By similar reasoning, Inacc is also related to sample cut-off or Q, and to predictive values (Sect. 2.3.1 and 2.3.2):

$$\text{Inacc} = (1 - \text{PPV} \cdot Q) + (1 - \text{NPV} \cdot Q')$$
$$= (\text{FDR} \cdot Q) + (\text{FRR} \cdot Q')$$

Worked Example: Inacc

In the screening test accuracy study of MACE [14], at the MACE cut-off of $\leq$20/30, TP = 104, FN = 10, FP = 188, and TN = 453.

Hence the value for Inacc at this cut-off is:

$$\text{Inacc} = (\text{FP} + \text{FN})/(\text{TP} + \text{FP} + \text{FN} + \text{TN})$$
$$= (188 + 10)/(104 + 188 + 10 + 453)$$
$$= 0.262$$

Inacc may also be expressed in terms of P, P', FNR and FPR. Values for the latter two terms at this MACE cut-off are 0.088 and 0.293 respectively (Sect. 2.2.2).

Hence the value for Inacc is:

$$\text{Inacc} = (\text{FNR} \cdot \text{P}) + (\text{FPR} \cdot \text{P}')$$
$$= (0.088 \times 0.151) + (0.293 \times 0.849)$$
$$= 0.262$$

Inacc may also be expressed in terms of Q, Q′, PPV and NPV. In the MACE study [14], Q = 0.387 and Q′ = 0.613 (Sect. 1.3.2). Values for PPV and NPV at this MACE cut-off are 0.356 and 0.978 respectively (Sect. 2.3.1).

Hence the value for Inacc is:

$$\text{Inacc} = (1 - \text{PPV} \cdot \text{Q}) + (1 - \text{NPV} \cdot \text{Q}')$$
$$= [(1-0.356) \times 0.387] + [(1-0.978) \times 0.613]$$
$$= 0.262$$

The reciprocal of Inacc has been defined as the "number needed to misdiagnose" (Sect. 5.5).

Acc and Inacc are scalar values based on information from both columns of the 2 × 2 table (cf. Sens and Spec), hence vary with prevalence, P (Sect. 2.3.3), as well as with the level of the test, Q, and hence with test cut-off [14, 17] (Fig. 3.4), and are also sensitive to class imbalance. Hence other forms of Acc and their complements may be calculated, including the balanced accuracy (Sect. 3.2.6), unbiased accuracy (Sect. 3.2.7), and quality accuracy (Sect. 6.2.3).

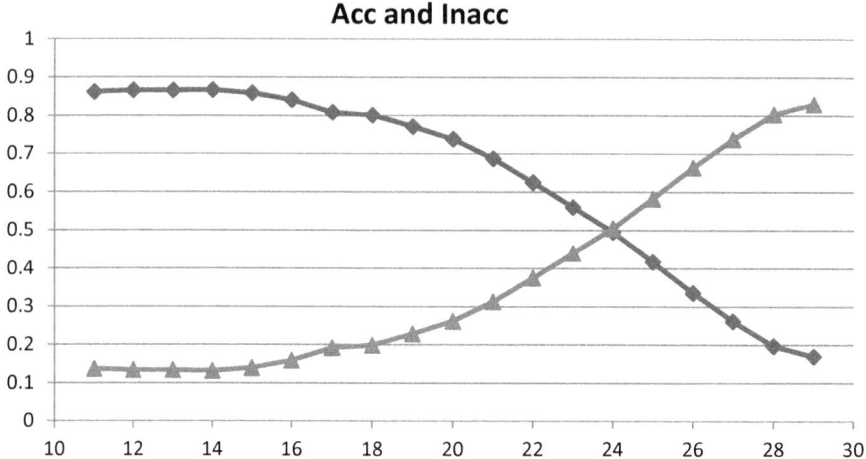

Fig. 3.4 Plot of accuracy (diamonds) and Inaccuracy (triangles) for dementia diagnosis at fixed P (= 0.151) on y axis versus MACE cut-off (x axis) (data from [14])

3.2.6 Balanced Accuracy and Inaccuracy (BAcc, BInacc)

As previously shown (Sect. 3.2.5):

$$Acc = (Sens \cdot P) + (Spec \cdot P')$$

Thus, in the particular case of a balanced dataset, where $P = P' = 0.5$, a "balanced accuracy" (BAcc) may be calculated [2, 3, 33], where:

$$BAcc = (Sens + Spec)/2$$

BAcc ranges from 0 to 1, with higher values better. Its complement is balanced inaccuracy (BInacc) [22]:

$$\begin{aligned} BInacc &= 1 - BAcc \\ &= [(1 - Sens) \cdot P] + \left[(1 - Spec) \cdot P'\right] \\ &= (FNR \cdot P) + (FPR \cdot P') \\ &= (FNR + FPR)/2 \end{aligned}$$

BAcc is best used where prevalence is far from 0.5 (i.e. where there is marked disparity between P and P') in order to avoid the high (and possibly over-optimistic) values of Acc which may occur when examining a biased classifier and/or an imbalanced dataset, consequent upon the weighting, in order to "pull" the value back to(wards) that of a balanced dataset (where $P = P' = 0.5$). When datasets are well-balanced, the values of Acc and Balanced Acc usually converge.

Worked Example: Balanced Accuracy (BAcc) and Balanced Inaccuracy (BInacc)

In the screening test accuracy study of MACE [14], at the MACE cut-off of $\leq$ 20/30, Sens $= 0.912$ and Spec $= 0.707$ (Sect. 2.2.1).
  Hence the value for BAcc at this MACE cut-off is:

$$\begin{aligned} BAcc &= (Sens + Spec)/2 \\ &= (0.912 + 0.707)/2 \\ &= 0.810 \end{aligned}$$

Note how this differs from the standard calculation of Acc at this cut-off ($=$ 0.738).

$$\begin{aligned} BInacc &= (FNR + FPR)/2 \\ &= (0.088 + 0.293)/2 \end{aligned}$$

$$= 0.190$$
$$= 1 - \text{BAcc}$$

Note how this differs from the standard calculation of Inacc at this cut-off (= 0.262).

BAcc may also be related to the Youden index (Y) (Sect. 4.2) and to the area under the receiver operating characteristic curve (AUC ROC) (Sect. 7.2.2).

Another form of "balanced accuracy" may also be calculated from predictive values (Sect. 3.3.3).

3.2.7 Unbiased Accuracy and Inaccuracy (UAcc, UInacc)

As discussed previously (Sect. 2.2.1), Sens and Spec are unscaled measures, and hence so is Acc. As an unscaled measure, it gives no direct measure of the degree to which diagnostic uncertainty is reduced. This can be addressed by calculating an unbiased accuracy (UAcc) which takes into account not only the value of P (Sect. 3.2.5) but also the value of Q, thus removing the biasing effects of random associations between test result and disease prevalence ([7], p.470), such that:

$$\text{UAcc} = \left(\text{Sens} \cdot P + \text{Spec} \cdot P'\right) - \left(P \cdot Q + P' \cdot Q'\right)/1 - \left(P \cdot Q + P' \cdot Q'\right)$$
$$= \text{Acc} - \left(P \cdot Q + P' \cdot Q'\right)/1 - \left(P \cdot Q + P' \cdot Q'\right)$$

UAcc has a range 0 to 1, where 0 = ineffective test and 1 = perfect test. Its complement is unbiased inaccuracy (UInacc = 1–UAcc) [22]. UAcc is equivalent to Cohen's kappa statistic (Sect. 8.4.2).

Worked Example: Unbiased Acc (UAcc) and Unbiased Inacc (UInacc)

In the screening test accuracy study of MACE [14], dementia prevalence (P) was 0.151. The positive sign rate, $Q = (TP + FP)/N$, was 0.387 (Sect. 1.3.2).

At the MACE cut-off of $\leq 20/30$, Sens = 0.912 and Spec = 0.707 (Sect. 2.2.1).

Hence the value for unbiased Acc at this MACE cut-off is:

$$\text{UAcc} = (\text{Sens} \cdot P + \text{Spec} \cdot P') - (P \cdot Q + P' \cdot Q')/1 - (P \cdot Q + P' \cdot Q')$$
$$= (0.138 + 0.600) - (0.058 + 0.520)/1 - (0.058 + 0.520)$$
$$= 0.738 - 0.579/1 - 0.579$$
$$= 0.159/0.421$$

$$= 0.378$$

Note how this differs from the calculation of Acc (= 0.738) and BAcc (0.810) at this cut-off.

$$\text{UInacc} = 1 - \text{UAcc}$$
$$= 1 - 0.378$$
$$= 0.622$$

Note how this differs from the values of Inacc (= 0.262) and BInacc (0.190) at this cut-off.

In the particular case of a balanced dataset, where $P = P' = 0.5$, then:

$$\text{UAcc} = 0.5(\text{Sens} + \text{Spec}) - 0.5(Q + Q')/1 - 0.5(Q + Q')$$

Since BAcc $= 0.5(\text{Sens} + \text{Spec})$ (Sect. 3.2.6) and $(Q + Q') = 1$ (Sect. 1.3.2), then:

$$\text{UAcc} = (\text{BAcc} - 0.5)/0.5$$
$$= 2.\text{BAcc} - 1$$

This is equivalent to the Youden index (Y; Sect. 4.2) and also the balanced identification index (BII; see Sect. 4.6.2) [22].

In the particular case where $Q = Q' = 0.5$, then:

$$\text{UAcc} = (\text{Sens} \cdot P + \text{Spec} \cdot P') - 0.5(P + P')/1 - 0.5(P + P')$$

Since Acc $= (\text{Sens.}P + \text{Spec. }P')$ (Sect. 3.2.5) and $(P + P') = 1$ (Sect. 1.3.2), then:

$$\text{UAcc} = \text{Acc} - 0.5/0.5$$
$$= 2.\text{Acc} - 1$$

This is equivalent to the identification index (II; see Sect. 4.6.1) [22].

Another method to scale accuracy is to use the quality measures for Sens and Spec to derive quality accuracy, QAcc (Sect. 6.2.3).

UAcc values, correcting for both P and Q, are extremely stringent; few tests have UAcc > 1 [22].

3.3   Information-Based Measures

3.3.1   Positive Predictive Value (PPV) and False Discovery Rate (FDR)

As previously shown (Sect. 2.3.2), false discovery rate (FDR) is the complement of positive predictive value (PPV):

$$FDR = (1 - PPV)$$

This is illustrated in the worked examples of PPV (Sect. 2.3.1) and FDR (Sect. 2.3.2) from the MACE study [14] showing that the calculated values (PPV = 0.356, FDR = 0.644) sum to 1. Hence knowing either PPV or FDR will always disclose the other across the range of test cut-offs (i.e. variation with Q; Fig. 3.5). This also holds for values rescaled according to Q [14, 15] (Sects. 6.3.1 and 6.3.2).

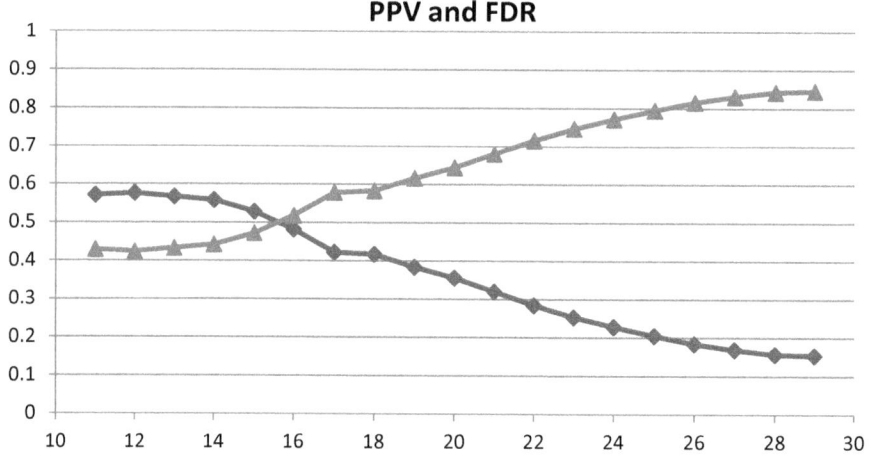

Fig. 3.5 Plot of PPV (diamonds) and FDR (triangles) for dementia diagnosis at fixed P (= 0.151) on y axis versus MACE cut-off (x axis) (data from [14])

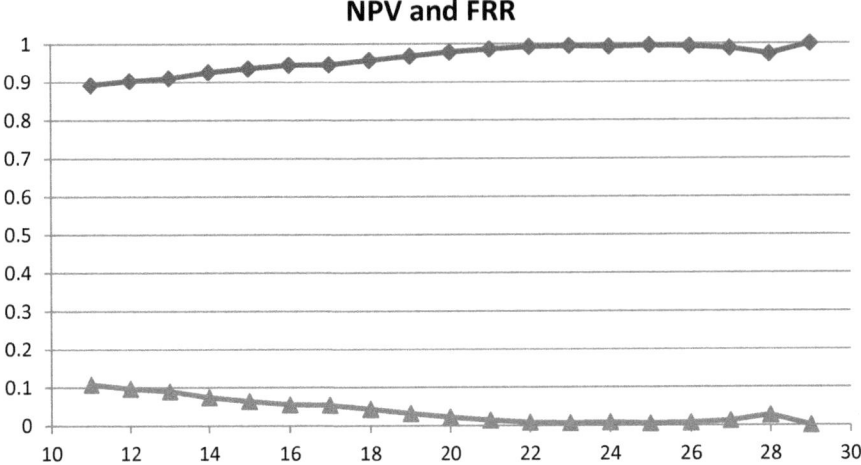

Fig. 3.6 Plot of NPV (diamonds) and FRR (triangles) for dementia diagnosis at fixed P (= 0.151) on y axis versus MACE cut-off (x axis) (data from [14])

3.3.2   Negative Predictive Value (NPV) and False Reassurance Rate (FRR)

As previously shown (Sect. 2.3.2), false reassurance rate (FRR) is the complement of negative predictive value (NPV):

$$FRR = (1 - NPV).$$

This is illustrated in the worked examples of NPV (Sect. 2.3.1) and FRR (Sect. 2.3.2) from the MACE study [14] showing that the calculated values (NPV = 0.978, FRR = 0.022) sum to 1. Hence knowing either NPV or FRR will always disclose the other across the range of test cut-offs (i.e. variation with Q; Fig. 3.6). This also holds for values rescaled according to Q [14, 15] (Sects. 6.3.1 and 6.3.2).

Note from Fig. 3.6 that this is the only example from the MACE study illustrated hitherto in this chapter in which there is no cross-over between the complementary measures plotted versus cut-off, i.e. the ideal of separation is achieved. Clearly this is a consequence of the skewed nature of the dataset in this particular study, with a very large number of true negatives and a very small number of false negatives (Fig. 2.2).

3.3.3 "Balanced Level" Formulations (BLAcc, BLInacc)

Just as it is possible to calculate balanced accuracy and inaccuracy from values of Sens, Spec, FNR and FPR (Sect. 3.2.6), one might also calculate a balanced measure related to the predictive values PPV, NPV, FDR and FRR. Because predictive values are related to the level of the test, Q (Sects. 1.3.2 and 2.3.4), I venture to call these "balanced level" formulations. Since:

$$\text{Sens} = \text{PPV} \cdot \text{Q/P}$$
$$\text{Spec} = \text{NPV} \cdot \text{Q}'/\text{P}'$$

and:

$$\text{Acc} = (\text{Sens} \cdot \text{P}) + (\text{Spec} \cdot \text{P}')$$
$$\text{Inacc} = (1 - \text{Sens}) \cdot \text{P} + (1 - \text{Spec}) \cdot \text{P}'$$

then substituting:

$$\text{Acc} = (\text{PPV} \cdot \text{Q}) + (\text{NPV} \cdot \text{Q}')$$
$$\text{Inacc} = (1 - \text{PPV}) \cdot \text{Q} + (1 - \text{NPV}) \cdot \text{Q}'$$
$$= (\text{FDR} \cdot \text{Q}) + (\text{FRR} \cdot \text{Q}')$$

In the particular case where Q = Q' = 0.5, both "balanced level accuracy" (BLAcc) and "balanced level inaccuracy" (BLInacc) values may be derived:

$$\text{BLAcc} = (\text{PPV} + \text{NPV})/2$$

$$\text{BLInacc} = 1 - \text{BLAcc}$$
$$= [(1 - \text{PPV}) + (1 - \text{NPV})]/2$$
$$= (\text{FDR} + \text{FRR})/2$$

Worked Examples: Balanced Level Accuracy (BLAcc) and Balanced Level Inaccuracy (BLInacc)

In the screening test accuracy study of MACE [14], at the MACE cut-off of ≤ 20/30, PPV = 0.356 and NPV = 0.978 (Sect. 2.3.1); FDR = 0.644 and FRR = 0.022 (Sect. 2.3.2).

Hence the values for BLAcc and BLInacc at this MACE cut-off are:

$$\text{BLAcc} = (\text{PPV} + \text{NPV})/2$$

$$= (0.356 + 0.978)/2$$
$$= 0.667$$

$$\text{BLInacc} = (\text{FDR} + \text{FRR})/2$$
$$= (0.644 + 0.022)/$$
$$= 0.333$$
$$= 1 - \text{BLAcc}$$

BLAcc may also be related to the predictive summary index (PSI) (Sect. 4.3).

3.4 Dependence of Paired Complementary Measures on Prevalence (P)

Having illustrated the dependence of the various paired measures on test cut-off (or Q) at a fixed prevalence (Figs. 3.2, 3.3, 3.4, 3.5 and 3.6), here their dependence on prevalence (P) at a fixed cut-off is shown.

Whilst choosing the fixed value of P may be straightforward (the base rate of the study population), choosing a fixed value of Q may not be so evident. Options include maximal test Acc, or maximal Youden index ([18], p.156–9 and 163–5). For the purposes of this illustration, maximal Youden index has been used (Sect. 4.2), which occurs at MACE cut-off $\leq$ 20/30.

Values for PPV and NPV may be calculated using Bayes' formula (Sect. 2.3.3):

$$\text{PPV} = \text{Sens} \times \text{P}/(\text{Sens} \times \text{P}) + \left[(1 - \text{Spec}) \times (1 - \text{P})\right]$$
$$= \text{Sens} \times \text{P}/(\text{Sens} \times \text{P}) + [\text{FPR} \times (1 - \text{P})]$$

$$\text{NPV} = \text{Spec} \times (1 - \text{P})/\left[\text{Spec} \times (1 - \text{P})\right] + [(1 - \text{Sens}) \times \text{P}]$$
$$= \text{Spec} \times (1 - \text{P})/\left[\text{Spec} \times (1 - \text{P})\right] + [\text{FNR} \times \text{P}]$$

FDR and FRR values are then the complements of PPV and NPV respectively. Values for Acc may be calculated using the equation (Sect. 3.2.5):

$$\text{Acc} = (\text{Sens} \cdot \text{P}) + \left(\text{Spec} \cdot \text{P}'\right)$$

At MACE cut-off $\leq$ 20/30, this simplifies to:

$$\text{Acc} = 0.912 \cdot \text{P} + 0.707 \cdot \text{P}'$$

Table 3.1 Values of Sens, FNR, Spec, and FPR for dementia diagnosis at fixed MACE cut-off of $\leq 20/30$ (= maximal Youden index; fixed $Q = 0.387$) at various prevalence levels

P, P'	Sens	FNR	Spec	FPR
0.1, 0.9	0.914	0.086	0.681	0.319
0.2, 0.8	0.908	0.092	0.728	0.272
0.3, 0.7	0.896	0.104	0.763	0.237
0.4, 0.6	0.884	0.116	0.790	0.210
0.5, 0.5	0.865	0.135	0.812	0.188
0.6, 0.4	0.840	0.160	0.830	0.170
0.7, 0.3	0.803	0.197	0.844	0.156
0.8, 0.2	0.746	0.254	0.857	0.143
0.9, 0.1	0.640	0.360	0.868	0.132

Inacc values are then the complements of Acc values.

Values for Sens and Spec at a fixed Q may be calculated using the equivalences defined by Kraemer [12]:

$$(\text{Sens} - Q)/Q' = (\text{NPV} - P')/P$$

and

$$(\text{Spec} - Q')/Q = (\text{PPV} - P)/P'$$

Hence:

$$\text{Sens} = [Q' \cdot (\text{NPV} - P')/P] + Q$$

and

$$\text{Spec} = [Q \cdot (\text{PPV} - P)/P'] + Q'$$

(These equations for Sens and Spec simplify to Sens = PPV.Q/P and Spec = NPV.Q'/P' as shown in Sect. 2.3.4).

FNR and FPR values are then the complements of Sens and Spec respectively.

Calculated values for Sens, FNR, Spec and FPR at 0.1 increments of P are shown in Table 3.1 and illustrated in Figs. 3.7 and 3.8. Similarly for values of Acc and Inacc in Table 3.2 and Fig. 3.9; and for PPV, FDR, NPV and FRR in Table 3.3 and Figs. 3.10 and 3.11.

Note in Figs. 3.7, 3.8 and 3.9 that there is no cross-over between the complementary measures plotted versus prevalence at the chosen MACE test cut-off, i.e. the ideal of separation is achieved, and that in Figs. 3.10 and 3.11 cross-over only occurs at very low and very high disease prevalence respectively.

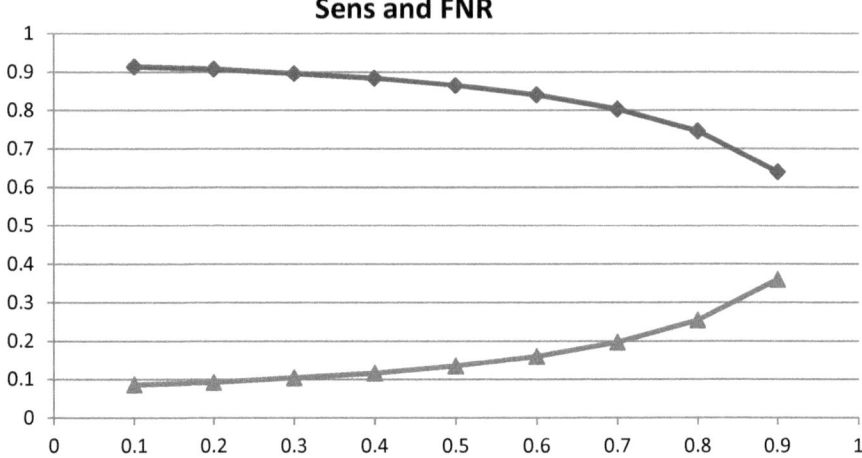

Fig. 3.7 Plot of sensitivity (diamonds) and FNR (triangles) for dementia diagnosis at fixed Q (= 0.387; MACE cut-off ≤ 20/30) on y axis versus prevalence P (x axis)

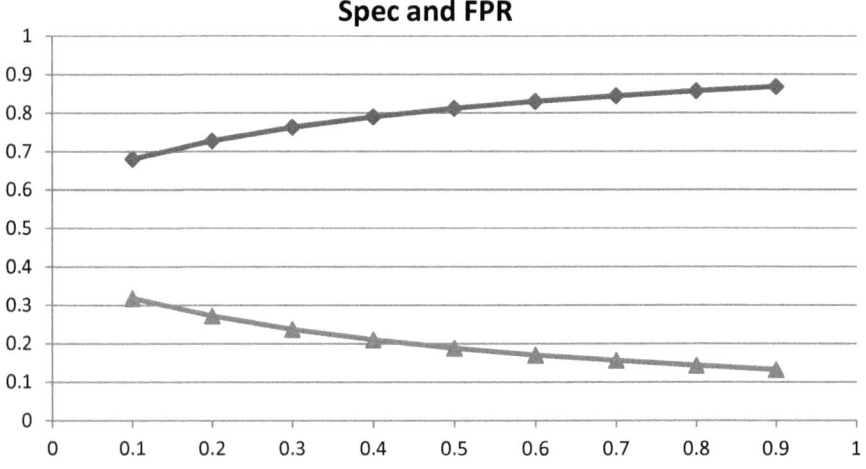

Fig. 3.8 Plot of specificity (diamonds) and FPR (triangles) for dementia diagnosis at fixed Q (= 0.387; MACE cut-off ≤ 20/30) on y axis versus prevalence P (x axis)

These plots suggest that for this test accuracy study of MACE, test Spec, Acc and PPV are better at high prevalence whereas Sens and NPV are better at low prevalence. This pattern is the converse of that seen with Q, with Spec, Acc and PPV better at lower cut-offs (compare Figs. 3.3, 3.4 and 3.5 with Figs. 3.8, 3.9 and 3.10 respectively) and Sens and NPV better at higher cut-offs (compare Figs. 3.2 and 3.6 with Figs. 3.7 and 3.11 respectively).

Table 3.2 Values of Acc and Inacc for dementia diagnosis at fixed MACE cut-off of ≤ 20/30 (= maximal Youden index; fixed Q = 0.387) at various prevalence levels

P, P′	Acc	Inacc
0.1, 0.9	0.728	0.272
0.2, 0.8	0.748	0.252
0.3, 0.7	0.769	0.231
0.4, 0.6	0.789	0.211
0.5, 0.5	0.810	0.190
0.6, 0.4	0.830	0.170
0.7, 0.3	0.851	0.149
0.8, 0.2	0.871	0.129
0.9, 0.1	0.892	0.108

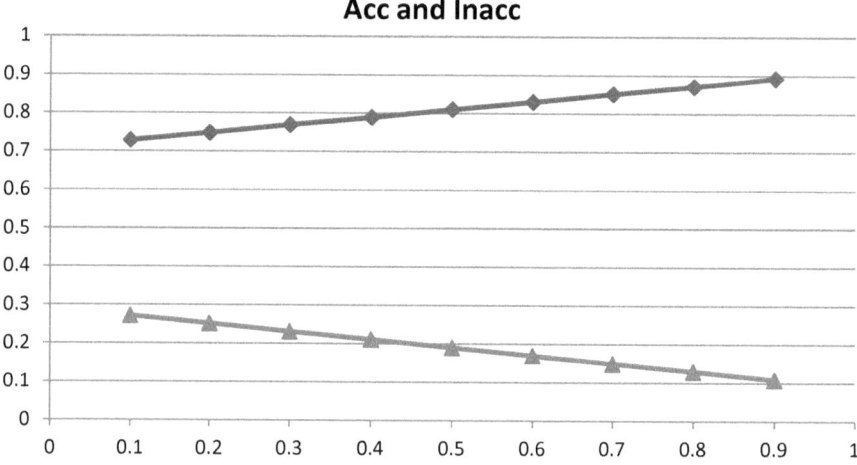

Fig. 3.9 Plot of accuracy (diamonds) and Inaccuracy (triangles) for dementia diagnosis at fixed Q (= 0.387; MACE cut-off ≤ 20/30) on y axis versus prevalence P (x axis)

Table 3.3 Values of PPV, FDR, NPV, and FRR for dementia diagnosis at fixed MACE cut-off of ≤20/30 (= maximal Youden index; fixed Q = 0.387) at various prevalence levels

P, P′	PPV	FDR	NPV	FRR
0.1, 0.9	0.257	0.743	0.986	0.014
0.2, 0.8	0.437	0.563	0.970	0.030
0.3, 0.7	0.571	0.429	0.949	0.051
0.4, 0.6	0.675	0.325	0.924	0.076
0.5, 0.5	0.757	0.243	0.890	0.110
0.6, 0.4	0.824	0.176	0.843	0.157
0.7, 0.3	0.879	0.121	0.775	0.225
0.8, 0.2	0.926	0.074	0.668	0.332
0.9, 0.1	0.966	0.034	0.472	0.528

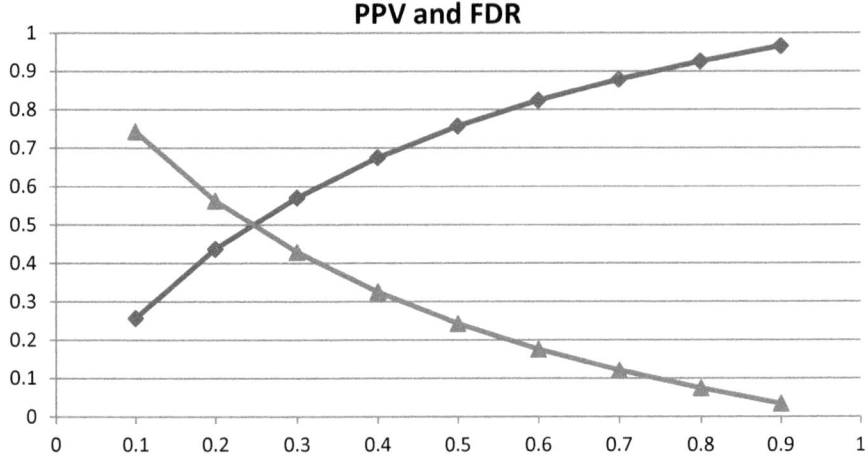

Fig. 3.10 Plot of PPV (diamonds) and FDR (triangles) for dementia diagnosis at fixed Q (= 0.387; MACE cut-off ≤ 20/30) on y axis versus prevalence P (x axis). Note equivalence of PPV curve to the conditional probability plot shown in Fig. 2.3

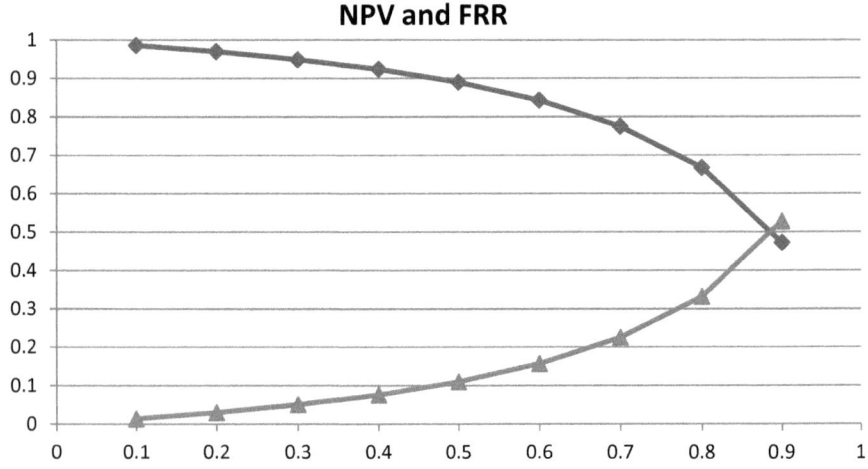

Fig. 3.11 Plot of NPV (diamonds) and FRR (triangles) for dementia diagnosis at fixed Q (= 0.387; MACE cut-off ≤20/30) on y axis versus prevalence P (x axis). Note equivalence of FRR curve to the conditional probability plot shown in Fig. 2.3

The interrelationship of P and Q may be illustrated by plotting a series of curves for different Q values against P. This is shown for Sens and Spec using the MACE dataset (Table 3.4, Figs. 3.12 and 3.13). At different selected MACE cut-offs (fixed values of Q and Q′) Sens and Spec were calculated (using the above equations) against variable P. Note that in this instance, PPV and NPV were also fixed for cut-off, and not recalculated for P (as in Table 3.1, Figs. 3.7 and 3.8). Again, the finding is that, for this test accuracy study of MACE, Sens improves with increasing Q as P increases, and conversely Spec decreases with increasing Q as P increases. These findings reflect the high sensitivity low specificity nature of MACE for dementia diagnosis [14]. Different findings may be anticipated with tests showing different performance characteristics (e.g. high sensitivity and high specificity, low sensitivity and high specificity).

Table 3.4 Interrelationship of P and Q illustrated using data from MACE study [14]

Cut-off	≤14/30	≤17/30	≤20/30	≤ 23/30	≤26/30
Q	0.159	0.264	0.387	0.585	0.812
Q′	0.841	0.736	0.613	0.415	0.188
PPV	0.558	0.422	0.356	0.253	0.184
NPV	0.926	0.946	0.978	0.994	0.993
Sens, Spec					
P, P′					
0.1, 0.9	0.378, 0.922	0.603, 0.830	0.865, 0.723	0.975, 0.514	0.986, 0.264
0.2, 0.8	0.689, 0.912	0.801, 0.809	0.933, 0.688	0.988, 0.454	0.993, 0.172
0.3, 0.7	0.793, 0.900	0.868, 0.782	0.955, 0.644	0.992, 0.376	0.996, 0.053
0.4, 0.6	0.844, 0.883	0.901, 0.746	0.966, 0.585	0.994, 0.272	0.997, −0.104
0.5, 0.5	0.876, 0.859	0.921, 0.695	0.973, 0.502	0.995, 0.126	0.997, −0.325
0.6, 0.4	0.896, 0.824	0.934, 0.619	0.978, 0.377	0.996, −0.09	0.998, −0.656
0.7, 0.3	0.911, 0.766	0.943, 0.491	0.981, 0.169	0.996, −0.457	0.998, −1.21
0.8, 0.2	0.922, 0.649	0.950, 0.237	0.983, −0.246	0.997, −1.18	0.998, −2.31
0.9, 0.1	0.931, 0.297	0.956, −0.526	0.985, −1.49	0.997, −3.37	0.999, −5.63

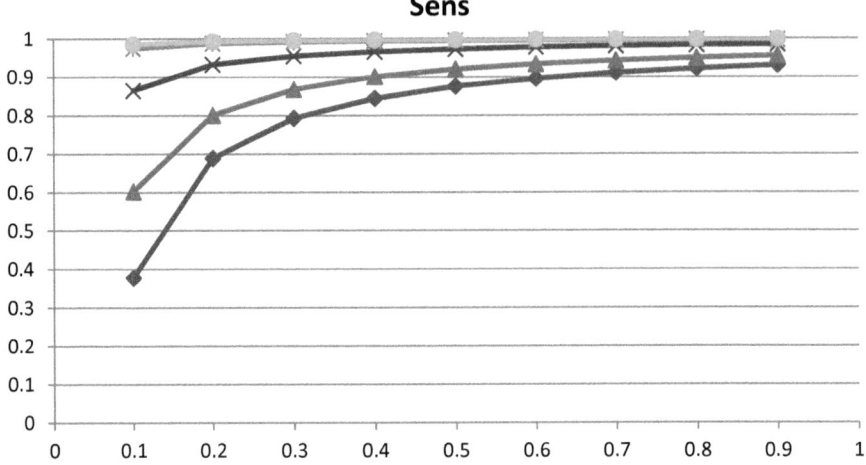

Fig. 3.12 Plot of Sens for five different MACE cut-offs (hence different values of Q) on y axis versus prevalence P (x axis); from data in Table 3.4

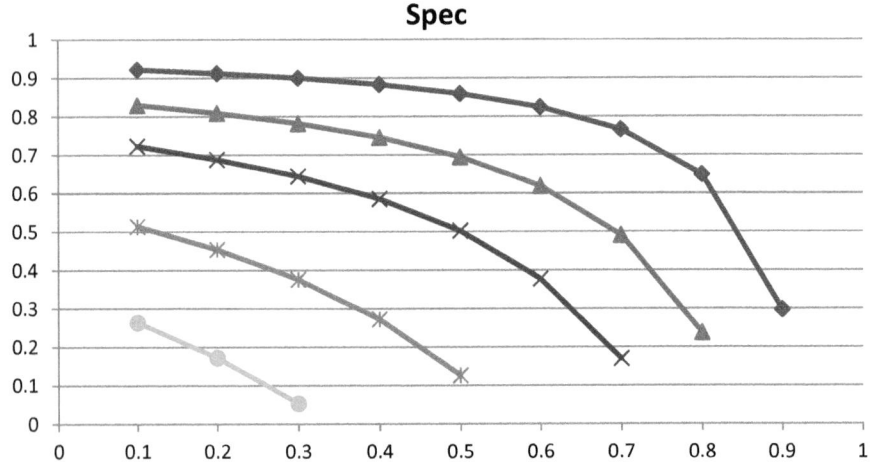

Fig. 3.13 Plot of Spec for five different MACE cut-offs (hence different values of Q) on y axis versus prevalence P (x axis); from data in Table 3.4

References

1. Bossuyt PMM. Clinical validity: defining biomarker performance. Scand J Clin Lab Invest. 2010;70(Suppl242):46–52.
2. Brodersen KH, Ong CS, Stephan KE, Buhmann JM. The balanced accuracy and its posterior distribution. In: Proceedings of ICPR 2010—the 20th IAPR International Conference on Pattern Recognition. Istanbul: IEEE, 2010:3121–4.

3. Chicco D, Tötsch N, Jurman G. The Matthews correlation coefficient (MCC) is more reliable than balanced accuracy, bookmaker informedness, and markedness in two-class confusion matrix evaluation. BioData Mining. 2021;14:13.
4. Connell FA, Koepsell TD. Measures of gain in certainty from a diagnostic test. Am J Epidemiol. 1985;121:744–53.
5. Freidson E. Profession of medicine. A study of the sociology of applied knowledge. New York: Dodd, Mead; [1970] 1975.
6. Gallagher EJ. The problem with sensitivity and specificity... Ann Emerg Med. 2003;42:298–303.
7. Garrett CT, Sell S. Summary and perspective: assessing test effectiveness—the identification of good tumour markers. In: Garrett CT, Sell S, editors. Cellular cancer markers. Springer; 1995. p. 455–77.
8. Habibzadeh F, Habibzadeh P, Yadollahie M. On determining the most appropriate test cut-off value: the case of tests with continuous results. Biochem Med (Zagreb). 2016;26:297–307.
9. Hancock P, Larner AJ. Clinical utility of Patient Health Questionnaire-9 (PHQ-9) in memory clinics. Int J Psychiatry Clin Pract. 2009;13:188–91.
10. Hsieh S, McGrory S, Leslie F, Dawson K, Ahmed S, Butler CR, et al. The Mini-Addenbrooke's Cognitive Examination: a new assessment tool for dementia. Dement Geriatr Cogn Disord. 2015;39:1–11.
11. Kaivanto K. Maximization of the sum of sensitivity and specificity as a diagnostic cutpoint criterion. J Cin Epidemiol. 2008;61:517–8.
12. Kraemer HC. Evaluating medical tests. Objective and quantitative guidelines. Newbery Park, California: Sage; 1992.
13. Larner AJ. Comparing diagnostic accuracy of cognitive screening instruments: a weighted comparison approach. Dement Geriatr Cogn Disord Extra. 2013;3:60–5.
14. Larner AJ. MACE for diagnosis of dementia and MCI: examining cut-offs and predictive values. Diagnostics (Basel). 2019;9:E51.
15. Larner AJ. Applying Kraemer's Q (positive sign rate): some implications for diagnostic test accuracy study results. Dement Geriatr Cogn Dis Extra. 2019;9:389–96.
16. Larner AJ. What is test accuracy? Comparing unitary accuracy metrics for cognitive screening instruments. Neurodegener Dis Manag. 2019;9:277–81.
17. Larner AJ. Defining "optimal" test cut-off using global test metrics: evidence from a cognitive screening instrument. Neurodegener Dis Manag. 2020;10:223–30.
18. Larner AJ. Manual of screeners for dementia. Pragmatic test accuracy studies. London: Springer; 2020.
19. Larner AJ. Cognitive screening instruments for dementia: comparing metrics of test limitation. Dement Neuropsychol. 2021;16:458–63.
20. Larner AJ. Re: Diagnostic reasoning: conditional probability plots illustrate "SnNOut" and SpPIn" rules. https://www.bmj.com/content/376/bmj-2021-064389/rr-0. (08 Feb 2022)
21. Larner AJ. Intracranial bruit: Charles Warlow's challenge revisited. Pract Neurol. 2022;22:79–81.
22. Larner AJ. Accuracy of cognitive screening instruments reconsidered: overall, balanced, or unbiased accuracy? Neurodegener Dis Manag. 2022;12:67–76.
23. Mallett S, Halligan S, Thompson M, Collins GS, Altman DG. Interpreting diagnostic accuracy studies for patient care. BMJ. 2012;345: e3999.
24. McCrea MA. Mild traumatic brain injury and postconcussion syndrome. The new evidence base for diagnosis and treatment. Oxford: Oxford University Press; 2008.
25. McKay RA. Patient Zero and the making of the AIDS epidemic. Chicago and London: University of Chicago Press; 2017.
26. Meador CK. The art and science of nondisease. N Engl J Med. 1965;272:92–5.
27. Metz CE. Basic principles of ROC analysis. Semin Nucl Med. 1978;8:283–98.
28. Moons KGM, Stijnen T, Michel BC, Büller HR, Van Es GA, Grobbee DE, Habbema DF. Application of treatment thresholds to diagnostic-test evaluation: an alternative to the comparison of areas under receiver operating characteristic curves. Med Decis Making. 1997;17:447–54.

29. Peirce CS. The numerical measure of the success of predictions. Science. 1884;4:453–4.
30. Perkins NJ, Schisterman EF. The inconsistency of "optimal" cutpoints obtained using two criteria based on the receiver operating characteristic curve. Am J Epidemiol. 2006;163:670–5.
31. Smits N. A note on Youden's J and its cost ratio. BMC Med Res Methodol. 2010;10:89.
32. Strauss SE, Glasziou P, Richardson WS, Haynes RB. Evidence-based medicine. How to practice and teach EBM. 5th edn. Edinburgh: Elsevier; 2019.
33. Velez DR, White BC, Motsinger AA, et al. A balanced accuracy function for epistasis modelling in imbalanced datasets using multifactor dimensionality reduction. Genet Epidemiol. 2007;31:306–15.
34. Youden WJ. Index for rating diagnostic tests. Cancer. 1950;3:32–5.

Chapter 4
Unitary Measures

Contents

4.1 Introduction

In addition to the paired test measures examined in Chaps. 2 and 3, there are also a number of global, single, or unitary measures which may be used to summarise the outcomes of a 2×2 contingency table. Accuracy (Sect. 3.2.5) and diagnostic odds ratio (Sect. 2.4.1) are sometimes used as global outcome measures, but these are in fact paired (with inaccuracy and error odds ratio, respectively, although both the latter measures are seldom used).

4.2   Youden Index (Y) or Statistic (J)

Youden [61] defined the Youden index (Y), or Youden J statistic, as:

$$Y = \text{Sens} + \text{Spec} - 1$$

This parameter had in fact been previously formulated, apparently unknown to Youden, as the "science of the method," by Charles Sanders Peirce (1839–1914) in 1884 [50], also sometimes known as the Peirce skill score.

Hence, the Youden index is a measure which attempts to combine information from both sensitivity (Sens) and specificity (Spec), as do likelihood ratios (Sect. 2.3.5) and correct classification rate (Sect. 3.2.4).

Values of Y may range from -1 to $+1$. However, most values of Y would be expected to fall within the range 0 (worthless, no diagnostic value) to 1 (perfect diagnostic value, no false positives or false negatives), with negative values occurring only if the test were misleading, i.e. the test result was negatively associated with the true diagnosis.

Y may be termed "informedness" or bookmaker informedness in the informatics literature [53]. It has also been characterised as the maximum proportional reduction in expected "regret" achieved by a test, i.e. the difference in outcome between the action taken and the best action that could, in retrospect, have been taken [16].

Y may also be expressed in terms of false positive rate (FPR) and false negative rate (FNR) (Sect. 2.2.2) as:

$$\begin{aligned}
Y &= \text{Sens} - (1 - \text{Spec}) \\
&= \text{Sens} - \text{FPR} \\
&= \text{TPR} - \text{FPR}
\end{aligned}$$

or

$$\begin{aligned}
Y &= \text{Spec} - (1 - \text{Sens}) \\
&= \text{Spec} - \text{FNR} \\
&= \text{TNR} - \text{FNR} \\
&= 1 - (\text{FPR} + \text{FNR})
\end{aligned}$$

Hence Y is the difference between the two positive rates (TPR – FPR) or between the two negative rates (TNR–FNR). The outcomes of the addition of the two true rates (TPR + TNR) and of the two false rates (FNR + FPR) as respectively the correct classification rate and the misclassification rate have previously been described (Sect. 3.2.4). Hence:

$$\begin{aligned}
Y &= \text{Sens} + \text{Spec} - 1 \\
&= \text{TPR} + \text{TNR} - 1
\end{aligned}$$

$$= \text{Correct classification rate} - 1$$

or

$$Y = 1 - (\text{FPR} + \text{FNR})$$
$$= 1 - \text{Misclassification rate}$$

Y is therefore the complement of the correct classification and misclassification rates (or the sum of the two false rates), with the end points of $+1$ and -1.

In literal notation (Fig. 1.1):

$$Y = [\text{TP}/(\text{TP} + \text{FN})] + [\text{TN}/(\text{FP} + \text{TN})] - 1$$
$$= [\text{TP}/\text{p}] + [\text{TP}/\text{p}'] - 1$$

Y may also be computed from the raw cell values from the 2×2 contingency table without first calculating Sens and Spec:

$$Y = [(\text{TP} \times \text{TN}) - (\text{FP} \times \text{FN})]/[(\text{TP} + \text{FN})(\text{FP} + \text{TN})]$$

In algebraic notation (Fig. 1.2):

$$Y = [a/(a + c) + [d/(b + d)] - 1$$

or, without first calculating Sens and Spec:

$$Y = (ad - bc)/[(a + c) \cdot (b + d)]$$

or, in terms of marginal totals (Sect. 1.3.1):

$$Y = (ad - bc)/(p \cdot p')$$

In error notation:

$$Y = (1 - \beta) + (1 - \alpha) - 1$$
$$= 1 - (\alpha + \beta)$$

Y can also be expressed in terms of likelihood ratios (Sect. 2.3.5):

$$Y = \text{Sens} + \text{Spec} - 1$$
$$= (\text{PLR} - 1) \times (1 - \text{Spec})$$
$$= (\text{PLR} - 1) \times \text{FPR}$$
$$= (1 - \text{NLR}) \times \text{Spec}$$
$$= (\text{PLR} - 1) \times (1 - \text{NLR})/(\text{PLR} - \text{NLR})$$

For the particular case of a single-threshold binary classifier, there is also a method to calculate Y from the area under the receiver operating characteristic (ROC) plot (see Sect. 7.2.2).

Worked Examples: Youden Index (Y)

The Mini-Addenbrooke's Cognitive Examination (MACE) [17] was subjected to a screening test accuracy study [23]. At the MACE cut-off of $\leq 20/30$, TP $= 104$, FN $= 10$, FP $= 188$, and TN $= 453$ (Fig. 2.2).

Hence the values for Sens and Spec are (Sect. 2.2.1):

$$Sens = TP/(TP + FN)$$
$$= 104/(104 + 10)$$
$$= 0.912$$

$$Spec = TN/(TN + FP)$$
$$= 453/(453 + 188)$$
$$= 0.707$$

Therefore the value for Y is:

$$Y = Sens + Spec - 1$$
$$= 0.912 + 0.707 - 1$$
$$= 0.619$$

Examining all test cut-offs, this was the cut-off giving the maximal value for Youden index for dementia diagnosis [23] (hence use of this cut-off in previous worked examples).

Y may also be calculated without first knowing Sens and Spec:

$$Y = [(TP \times TN) - (FP \times FN)]/[(TP + FN)(FP + TN)]$$
$$= [(104 \times 453) - (188 \times 10)]/[(104 + 10)(188 + 453)]$$
$$= 45232/73074$$
$$= 0.619$$

It was previously shown (Sect. 2.3.5) that PLR $= 3.11$ and NLR $= 0.124$ at MACE cut-off $\leq 20/30$. Expressing Y in terms of LRs:

$$Y = (PLR - 1) \times (1 - NLR)/(PLR - NLR)$$
$$= (3.11 - 1) \times (1 - 0.124)/(3.11 - 0.124)$$

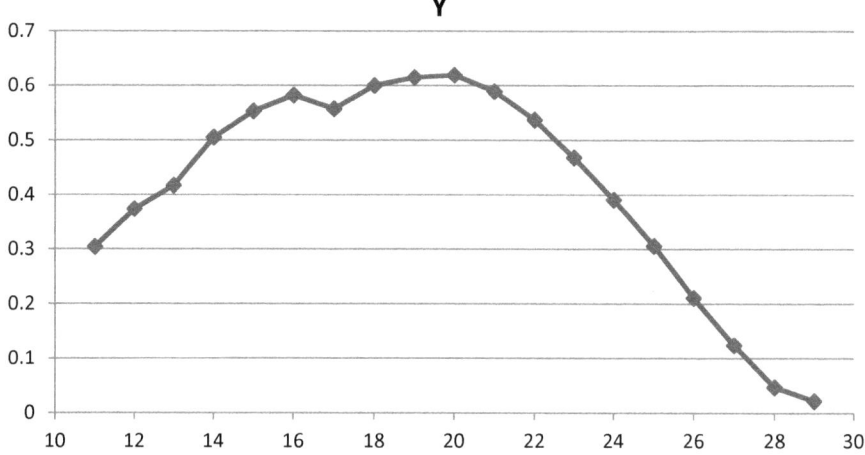

Fig. 4.1 Plot of Youden index (y axis) for dementia diagnosis at fixed P (= 0.151) versus MACE cut-off (x axis) [27]

$$= 2.11 \times 0.876/2.986$$
$$= 0.619$$

It was also previously shown (Sect. 3.2.4) that Correct classification rate was 1.619, hence Y = Correct classification rate −1.

It was also shown (Sect. 3.2.4) that Misclassification rate was 0.381, hence Y = 1−Misclassification rate.

Y varies with test cut-off (Fig. 4.1) [23, 27] and hence with Q. A rescaled quality Y may also be calculated [25] (Sect. 6.5.1).

As Y is dependent on P and Q, it may be expressed in terms of P, Q, and Sens, as [54]:

$$Y = (\text{Sens} - Q)/P'$$

Worked Example: Youden Index (Y)

In the MACE screening test accuracy study with P = 0.151 [23], at the MACE cut-off of ≤ 20/30, Q = 0.387 and Sens = 0.912.

Hence the value for Y is:

$$Y = (\text{Sens} - Q)/P'$$

Table 4.1 Values of Sens, Spec (from Table 3.1), and Y for dementia diagnosis at fixed MACE cut-off of ≤ 20/30 at various prevalence levels

P, P′	Sens	Spec	Y
0.1, 0.9	0.914	0.681	0.595
0.2, 0.8	0.908	0.728	0.636
0.3, 0.7	0.896	0.763	0.659
0.4, 0.6	0.884	0.790	0.674
0.5, 0.5	0.865	0.812	0.677
0.6, 0.4	0.840	0.830	0.670
0.7, 0.3	0.803	0.844	0.647
0.8, 0.2	0.746	0.857	0.603
0.9, 0.1	0.640	0.868	0.508

$$= (0.912 - 0.387)/0.849$$
$$= 0.619$$

Y has some shortcomings as a global measure [24]. Being derived from Sens and Spec, both strict columnar ratios, it would be anticipated that Y, like Sens and Spec, is independent of prevalence. Certainly Youden ([61], p.33) stated that Y was independent of the size, relative or absolute, of the control and disease groups. In practice, Sens and Spec, and hence Y, are not independent of disease prevalence [3], as is shown for the MACE study in Table 4.1 and Fig. 4.2 which indicate that in this dataset Y is optimal at $P = 0.5$. Moreover, Y implicitly employs a ratio of misclassification costs for FN and FP which varies with prevalence and so Y is not truly optimal [58]. Its maximal value arbitrarily assumes disease prevalence to be 50%, and treats FN and FP as equally undesirable, which is often not the case in clinical practice. In terms of cost ratio (Sect. 3.2.4), Y assumes $Cr = 0.5$, i.e. that the difference in costs between correct and incorrect test classification is equal for both the healthy and diseased [58].

Y may also be related to one of the formulations of Accuracy, specifically Balanced Accuracy (BAcc; Sect. 3.2.6) [35]. Since:

$$BAcc = (Sens + Spec)/2$$

and:

$$Y = Sens + Spec - 1$$

then:

$$Y + 1 = Sens + Spec$$

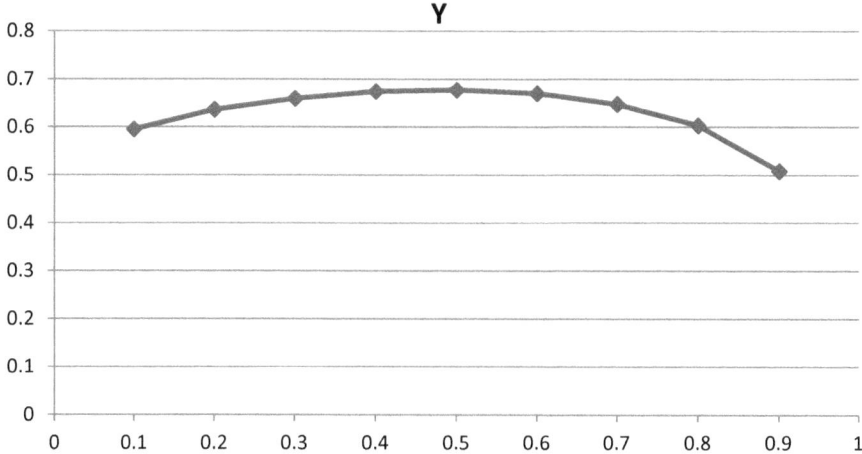

Fig. 4.2 Plot of Youden index (y axis) for dementia diagnosis at fixed Q (MACE cut-off ≤ 20/30) versus prevalence P (x axis)

Substituting:

$$BAcc = (Y + 1)/2$$

and rearranging:

$$Y = 2 \cdot BAcc - 1$$

Y also has an application in defining optimal test cut-off from the receiver operating characteristic (ROC) curve (Sect. 7.3.1) [1, 57].

The reciprocal (multiplicative inverse) of Y has been termed the number needed to diagnose (NND) [40] (see Sect. 5.2).

4.3 Predictive Summary Index (PSI, Ψ)

Linn and Grunau [40] defined the predictive summary index (PSI, Ψ), combining positive and negative predictive values (Sect. 2.3.1), as:

$$PSI = PPV + NPV - 1$$

Values of PSI may range from − 1 to + 1. However, most values of PSI would be expected to fall within the range 0 (no diagnostic value) to 1 (perfect predictive value, no false discoveries or false reassurances), with negative values occurring only if the test were misleading, i.e. the test result was negatively associated with the true diagnosis. PSI may be termed "markedness" or bookmaker markedness in the informatics literature [53].

PSI may also be expressed in terms of false discovery rate (FDR) and false reassurance rate (FRR) (Sect. 2.3.2) as:

$$\begin{aligned} \text{PSI} &= \text{PPV} - (1 - \text{NPV}) \\ &= \text{PPV} - \text{FRR} \\ &= \text{NPV} - (1 - \text{PPV}) \\ &= \text{NPV} - \text{FDR} \end{aligned}$$

This measure may be characterised as the net gain of certainty of a test, by summing gain in certainty that a condition is either present or absent:

$$\begin{aligned} \text{PSI} &= (\text{PPV} - \text{P}) + [\text{NPV} - (1 - \text{P})] \\ &= \text{PPV} + \text{NPV} - 1 \end{aligned}$$

In literal notation (Fig. 1.1):

$$\begin{aligned} \text{PSI} &= [\text{TP}/(\text{TP} + \text{FP})] + [\text{TN}/(\text{FN} + \text{TN})] - 1 \\ &= \left[\text{TP}/q\right] + \left[\text{TN}/q'\right] - 1 \end{aligned}$$

In algebraic notation (Fig. 1.2):

$$\text{PSI} = [a/(a + b)] + [d/(c + d)] - 1$$

PSI may also be computed from the raw cell values from the 2×2 contingency table without first calculating PPV and NPV:

$$\text{PSI} = [(\text{TP} \times \text{TN})] - (\text{FP} \times \text{FN})/[(\text{TP} + \text{FP})(\text{FN} + \text{TN})]$$

In algebraic notation:

$$\text{PSI} = (ad - bc)/[(a + b) \cdot (c + d)]$$

and in terms of marginal totals:

$$\text{PSI} = (ad - bc)/\left(q \cdot q'\right)$$

Worked Examples: Predictive Summary Index (PSI or Ψ)

In a screening test accuracy study of MACE [23], at the MACE cut-off giving maximal Youden index for dementia diagnosis, $\leq 20/30$, TP $= 104$, FN $= 10$, FP $= 188$, and TN $= 453$.

Hence the values for PPV and NPV at this cut-off are (Sect. 2.3.1):

$$PPV = TP/(TP + FP)$$
$$= 104/(104 + 188)$$
$$= 0.356$$

$$NPV = TN/(TN + FN)$$
$$= 453/(453 + 10)$$
$$= 0.978$$

Therefore the value for PSI is:

$$PSI = PPV + NPV - 1$$
$$= 0.356 + 0.978 - 1$$
$$= 0.334$$

PSI may also be calculated without first knowing PPV and NPV:

$$PSI = [(TP \times TN) - (FP \times FN)]/[(TP + FP)(FN + TN)]$$
$$= [(104 \times 453) - (188 \times 10)]/[(104 + 188)(10 + 453)]$$
$$= 45232/135196$$
$$= 0.334$$

PSI varies with test cut-off or Q (Fig. 4.3) [23], with a different maximal cut-off value from Y. Hence, a rescaled quality PSI, QPSI, may also be calculated [25] (Sect. 6.5.2).

PSI also varies with prevalence, as shown for the MACE study in Table 4.2 and Fig. 4.4, with optimal PSI at P $= 0.6$ (cf. Y, optimal at P $= 0.5$).

As PSI is dependent on P and Q, it may be expressed in terms of P, Q, and PPV as [54]:

$$PSI = (PPV - P)/Q'$$

PSI may also be expressed in terms of P, Q, and Y (since PPV and NPV may be expressed in terms of Sens, Spec, P and Q; Sect. 2.3.4) [6]:

$$PSI = \left(P - P^2/Q - Q^2\right) \cdot Y$$

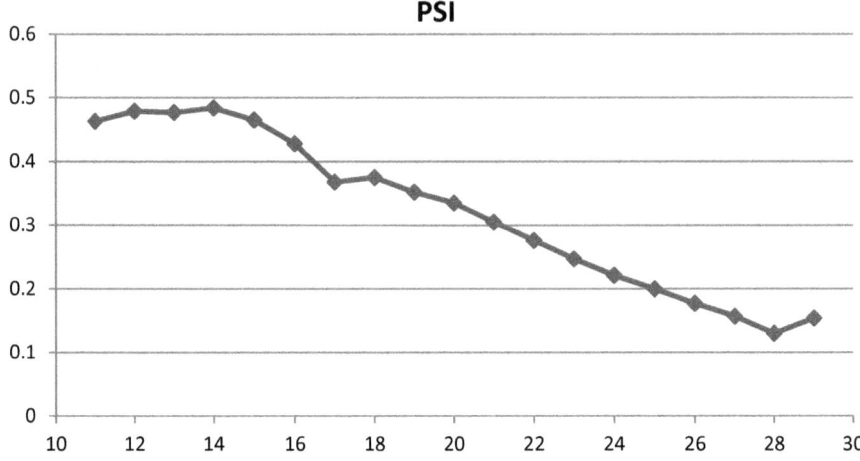

Fig. 4.3 Plot of PSI (y axis) for dementia diagnosis at fixed P (= 0.151) versus MACE cut-off (x axis) (data from [23])

Table 4.2 Values of PPV, NPV (from Table 3.3), and PSI for dementia diagnosis at fixed MACE cut-off of $\leq$ 20/30 at various prevalence levels

P, P′	PPV	NPV	PSI
0.1, 0.9	0.257	0.986	0.243
0.2, 0.8	0.437	0.970	0.407
0.3, 0.7	0.571	0.949	0.520
0.4, 0.6	0.675	0.924	0.599
0.5, 0.5	0.757	0.890	0.647
0.6, 0.4	0.824	0.843	0.667
0.7, 0.3	0.879	0.775	0.654
0.8, 0.2	0.926	0.668	0.594
0.9, 0.1	0.966	0.472	0.438

Worked Example: PSI Expressed in Terms of P, Q, PPV, and Y

In a screening test accuracy study of MACE [23], where P = 0.151 and the MACE cut-off $\leq$ 20/30 gave Q = 0.387 and Q′ = 0.613 (Sect. 1.3.2), PPV = 0.356 (Sect. 2.3.1), and Y = 0.619 (Sect. 4.2).

Hence using these figures:

$$PSI = (PPV - P)/Q'$$
$$= (0.356 - 0.151)/0.613$$
$$= 0.334$$

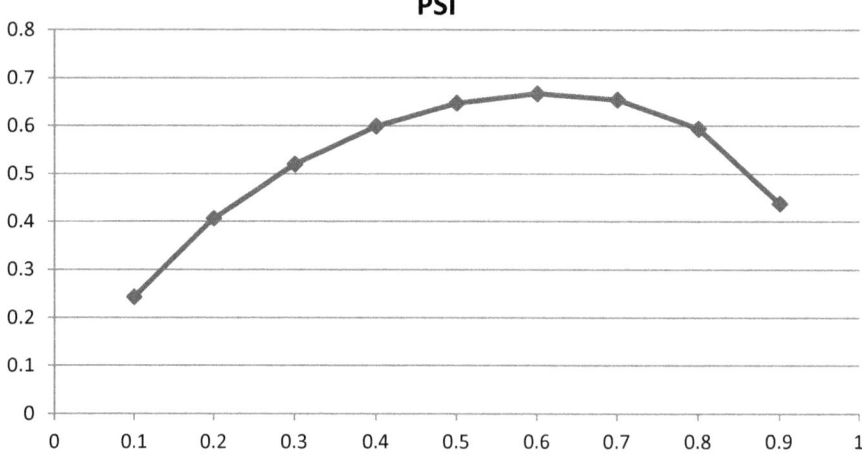

Fig. 4.4 Plot of PSI (y axis) for dementia diagnosis at fixed Q (MACE cut-off $\leq 20/30$) on versus prevalence P (x axis)

$$PSI = \left(P - P^2/Q - Q^2\right) \cdot Y$$
$$= (0.128/0.237) \cdot 0.619$$
$$= 0.334$$

PSI may also be related to the formulation of Balanced Level Accuracy (BLAcc) (Sect. 3.3.3) Since:

$$BLAcc = (PPV + NPV)/2$$

and:

$$PSI = PPV + NPV - 1$$

then:

$$PSI + 1 = PPV + NPV$$

Substituting:

$$BLAcc = (PSI + 1)/2$$

and rearranging:

$$PSI = 2 \cdot BLAcc - 1$$

Worked Example: PSI Expressed in Terms of Balanced Level Accuracy (BLAcc)

In the screening test accuracy study of MACE [23], at the MACE cut-off of $\leq$ 20/30, PPV = 0.356 and NPV = 0.978 (Sect. 2.3.1).

Hence the value for BLAcc at this MACE cut-off (Sect. 3.3.3) is:

$$BLAcc = (PPV + NPV)/2$$
$$= (0.356 + 0.978)/2$$
$$= 0.667$$

$$PSI = 2 \cdot BLAcc - 1$$
$$= (2 \times 0.667) - 1$$
$$= 0.334$$

It has been argued that PSI may be useful for making population-based policy decisions, but that it adds little useful information to practising clinicians attempting to apply research findings to individual patients [15].

The reciprocal (multiplicative inverse) of PSI has been termed the number needed to predict (NNP) [40] (see Sect. 5.3).

4.4   Harmonic Mean of Y and PSI (HMYPSI)

Just as Youden's index (Y) is an attempt to combine information about Sens and Spec, as are likelihood ratios (Sect. 2.3.5) and the receiver operating characteristic (ROC) curve (Sect. 7.2), and as predictive summary index (PSI) is an attempt to combine information about predictive values, it may also be helpful to have measures which attempt to combine Sens and Spec and predictive values. Options include the clinical utility indexes (Sect. 2.4.2) and the summary utility index (Sect. 4.9).

Another option is the mean of Y and PSI, either geometric, which is the Matthews' correlation coefficient (MCC; Sect. 4.5), or harmonic, since geometric and harmonic means have advantages over the arithmetic mean in skewed datasets. The "harmonic mean of Y and PSI" or HMYPSI (first described as such in [33], p.78–81) is given by:

$$HMYPSI = 2/[1/Y + 1/PSI]$$
$$= 2 \cdot Y \cdot PSI/(Y + PSI)$$

Like Y and PSI, the value of HMYPSI may range from -1 to $+1$, with higher values better.

Worked Example: Harmonic Mean of Y and PSI (HMYPSI)

In the screening test accuracy study of MACE [23], at the MACE cut-off of $\leq$ 20/30 the value of $Y = 0.619$ (Sect. 4.2) and of $PSI = 0.334$ (Sect. 4.3).

$$HMYPSI = 2.Y.PSI/(Y + PSI)$$
$$= 2 \times 0.619 \times 0.334/(0.619 + 0.334)$$
$$= 0.413/0.953$$
$$= 0.433$$

HMYPSI values vary with test cut-off or Q (Fig. 4.5), with maximal cut-off closer to that of PSI than to that of Y. A rescaled quality HMYPSI may be calculated (Sect. 6.5.3).

HMYPSI values also vary with prevalence (Table 4.3, Fig. 4.6).

Since HMYPSI is dependent on P and Q, it may be expressed in terms of P, Q, and either Y or PSI. As it is known (Sect. 4.3) that:

$$PSI = \left(P - P^2/Q - Q^2\right) \cdot Y$$

and:

$$HMYPSI = 2/[1/Y + 1/PSI]$$

Then substituting and rearranging:

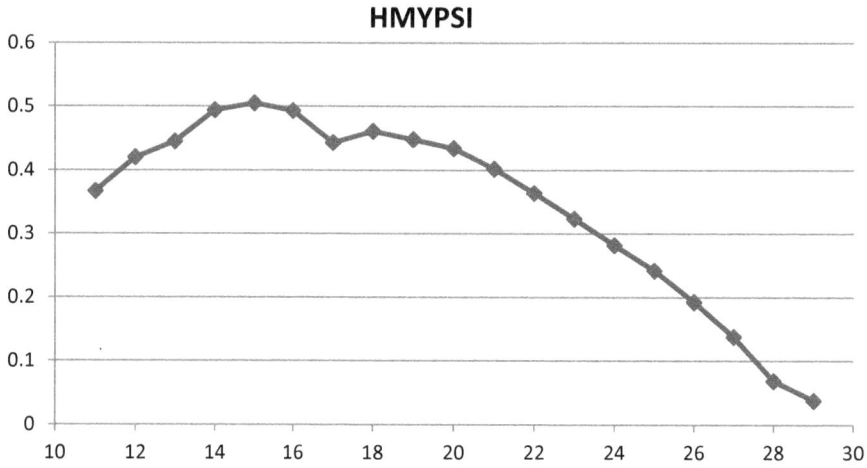

HMYPSI

Fig. 4.5 Plot of HMYPSI (y axis) for dementia diagnosis at fixed P ($= 0.151$) versus MACE cut-off (x axis)

Table 4.3 Values of Y (from Table 4.1), PSI (from Table 4.2), HMYPSI and MCC for dementia diagnosis at fixed MACE cut-off of ≤20/30 at various prevalence levels

P, P'	Y	PSI	HMYPSI	MCC
0.1, 0.9	0.595	0.243	0.345	0.380
0.2, 0.8	0.636	0.407	0.496	0.509
0.3, 0.7	0.659	0.520	0.581	0.585
0.4, 0.6	0.674	0.599	0.634	0.635
0.5, 0.5	0.677	0.647	0.662	0.662
0.6, 0.4	0.670	0.667	0.668	0.668
0.7, 0.3	0.647	0.654	0.650	0.650
0.8, 0.2	0.603	0.594	0.598	0.598
0.9, 0.1	0.508	0.438	0.470	0.472

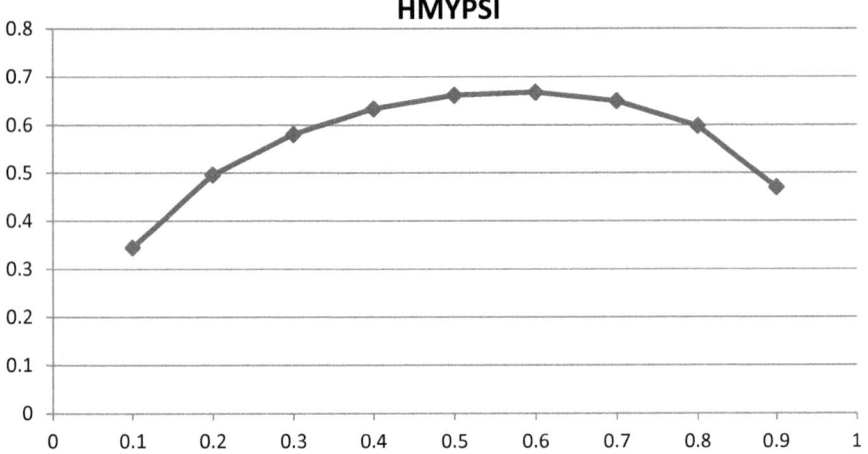

Fig. 4.6 Plot of HMYPSI (y axis) for dementia diagnosis at fixed Q (MACE cut-off ≤20/30) versus prevalence P (x axis)

$$\mathrm{HMYPSI} = 2/(1/\mathrm{Y}) \cdot \left[\left(1 + \left(\mathrm{Q} - \mathrm{Q}^2 \right) / \left(\mathrm{P} - \mathrm{P}^2 \right) \right) \right]$$

Similarly, since $\mathrm{Y} = \mathrm{PSI}/\left[\left(\mathrm{P} - \mathrm{P}^2 \right) / \left(\mathrm{Q} - \mathrm{Q}^2 \right) \right]$, then:

$$\mathrm{HMYPSI} = 2/(1/\mathrm{PSI}) \cdot \left[\left(\mathrm{P} - \mathrm{P}^2 \right) / \left(\mathrm{Q} - \mathrm{Q}^2 \right) + 1 \right]$$

Worked Examples: HMYPSI Expressed in Terms of P, Q, and Either Y or PSI

In a screening test accuracy study of MACE [23], where $P = 0.151$ and the MACE cut-off $\leq 20/30$ gave $Q = 0.387$ (Sect. 1.3.2), $Y = 0.619$ (Sect. 4.2), and $PSI = 0.334$ (Sect. 4.3).

Hence using these figures:

$$HMYPSI = 2/(1/Y) \cdot \left[\left(1 + (Q - Q^2)/(P - P^2)\right)\right]$$
$$= 2/(1/0.619) \cdot [1 + (0.237/0.128)]$$
$$= 0.433$$

$$HMYPSI = 2/(1/PSI) \cdot \left[\left(P - P^2\right)/\left(Q - Q^2\right) + 1\right]$$
$$= 2/(1/0.334) \cdot [(0.128/0.237) + 1]$$
$$= 0.433$$

In one particular case, when $b = c$ in the 2×2 contingency table (Fig. 1.2; i.e. false positives $=$ false negatives), and hence the marginal totals align (i.e. the matrix is symmetric), such that $(a + b) = (a + c)$ and $(b + d) = (c + d)$, then the values of HMYPSI and MCC coincide (in terms of marginal totals, when $p = q$ and $p' = q'$). In this situation, HMYPSI would also coincide with the value of the kappa statistic (Sect. 8.4.2).

4.5 Matthews' Correlation Coefficient (MCC)

Matthews [41] defined a correlation coefficient (MCC).

In literal notation:

$$MCC = [(TP \times TN) - (FP \times FN)]/\sqrt{[(TP + FP)(TP + FN)(TN + FP)(TN + FN)]}$$

In algebraic notation:

$$MCC = [(a \times d) - (b \times c)]/\sqrt{[(a + b) \cdot (a + c) \cdot (b + d) \cdot (c + d)]}$$
$$= (ad - bc)/\sqrt{(q \cdot p \cdot p' \cdot q')}$$

MCC is equivalent to the Pearson phi (φ) coefficient, an effect size from the family of measures of association (Sect. 8.3).

MCC is also the geometric mean of the Youden index (Y) or informedness (Sect. 4.2) and the predictive summary index (PSI) or markedness (Sect. 4.3):

$$MCC = \sqrt{(Y \times PSI)}$$

For those geometrically minded, calculation of MCC may be related to a theorem in elementary geometry: for a right triangle, ABC, the perpendicular AD divides BC into two portions, BD and DC. The length of the perpendicular $AD = \sqrt{(BD \times DC)}$, the geometric mean of BD and DC. If we substitute Y and PSI for BD and DC, then $AD = MCC$. The geometric mean is preferred to the arithmetic mean in skewed datasets, as is the harmonic mean (Sect. 4.4).

MCC has a range of -1 to $+1$, where $+1$ represents perfect prediction, 0 is no better than random, and -1 indicates total disagreement between prediction and observation.

A normalised MCC (nMCC), with range 0 to 1, may be calculated [5], for ease of comparison with other accuracy measures (e.g. [35]), as:

$$nMCC = (MCC + 1)/2$$

Worked Examples: Matthew's Correlation Coefficient (MCC)

In a screening test accuracy study of the MACE in a cohort of 755 consecutive patients [23], at the cut-off for dementia diagnosis of $\leq 20/30$, TP $= 104$, FN $= 10$, FP $= 188$, and TN $= 453$.

Hence the value for MCC is:

$$
\begin{aligned}
MCC &= [(TP \times TN) - (FP \times FN)]/\sqrt{[(TP + FP)(TP + FN)(TN + FP)(TN + FN)]} \\
&= [(104 \times 453) - (188 \times 10)]/\sqrt{[(104 + 188)(104 + 10)(188 + 453)(10 + 453)]} \\
&= 45232/99394.73 \\
&= 0.455
\end{aligned}
$$

It was previously shown for MACE at this cut-off that $Y = 0.619$ (Sect. 4.2) and $PSI = 0.334$ (Sect. 4.3).

Hence the value for MCC may also be calculated as:

$$
\begin{aligned}
MCC &= \sqrt{(Y \times PSI)} \\
&= \sqrt{(0.619 \times 0.334)} \\
&= 0.455
\end{aligned}
$$

The value for nMCC is:

$$nMCC = (MCC + 1)/2$$
$$= (0.455 + 1)/2$$
$$= 0.727$$

MCC values vary with test cut-off [27] in a pattern almost identical to that shown for HMYPSI (Fig. 4.5), with the same maximal cut-off (Table 7.2). Likewise, the variation of MCC with prevalence is almost identical to that for HMYPSI (Table 4.3), diverging only at the extremes. MCC may be expressed in terms of P, Q, and either Y or PSI [6]:

$$MCC = \sqrt{(P - P^2/Q - Q^2) \cdot Y}$$
$$= \sqrt{(Q - Q^2/P - P^2) \cdot PSI}$$

Worked Examples: MCC Expressed in Terms of P, Q, and Either Y or PSI

In a screening test accuracy study of MACE [23], where $P = 0.151$ and the MACE cut-off $\leq 20/30$ gave $Q = 0.387$ (Sect. 1.3.2), $Y = 0.619$ (Sect. 4.2), and $PSI = 0.334$ (Sect. 4.3).

Hence using these figures:

$$MCC = \sqrt{(P - P^2/Q - Q^2) \cdot Y}$$
$$= \sqrt{(0.128/0.237) \cdot 0.619}$$
$$= 0.455$$

$$MCC = \sqrt{(Q - Q^2/P - P^2) \cdot PSI}$$
$$= \sqrt{(0.237/0.128) \cdot 0.334}$$
$$= 0.455$$

A rescaled quality MCC may also be calculated (Sect. 6.5.4).

MCC is widely regarded as being a very informative score for establishing the quality of a binary classifier, since it takes into account the size of all four classes in the table, and allows for imbalanced data [2, 4, 5]. Hence it may be preferred to F measure (Sect. 4.8.3) [5]. MCC values have been calculated for several cognitive screening instruments and appear to be the least optimistic compared to Acc, area under the receiver operating characteristic curve (AUC ROC), and the F measure [26].

4.6 Identification Indexes

4.6.1 Identification Index (II)

Mitchell [47] proposed an identification index (II) based on Acc and Inacc (Sect. 3.2.5):

$$II = Acc - Inacc$$
$$= Acc - (1 - Acc)$$
$$= 2 \cdot Acc - 1$$

As Acc ranges from 0 to 1, and is the complement of Inacc (Sect. 3.2.5), II has a range of -1 to $+1$, with most scores anticipated in the range 0 to $+1$. A possible problem with II is that its value will be negative if Acc < 0.5.

In literal notation:

$$II = 2[(TP + TN)/(TP + FP + FN + TN)] - 1$$
$$= 2[(TP + TN)/N] - 1$$

In algebraic notation:

$$II = 2[(a + d)/(a + b + c + d)] - 1$$
$$= 2[(a + d)/N] - 1$$

In terms of marginal totals:

$$II = 2(r/N) - 1$$

Worked Example: Identification Index (II)

In a screening test accuracy study of MACE [23], at the MACE cut-off giving maximal Youden index for dementia diagnosis, $\leq 20/30$, TP $= 104$, FN $= 10$, FP $= 188$, and TN $= 453$.

Hence the value for Acc (Sect. 3.2.5) at this cut-off is:

$$Acc = (TP + TN)/(TP + FN + FP + TN)$$
$$= (104 + 453)/(104 + 10 + 188 + 453)$$
$$= 0.738$$

Therefore the value for II is:

$$II = 2 \cdot Acc - 1$$
$$= (2 \times 0.738) - 1$$
$$= 0.475$$

Acc and, hence, II both vary with the chosen test cut-off [23].

The original II formulation has been rarely adopted or examined [23, 28, 46]. Mendez called it the "Adjusted (for guessing) recognition score" ([46], p.88).

A rescaled quality II, QII, may be calculated (Sect. 6.5.5). The reciprocal (multiplicative inverse) of II has been termed the number needed to screen (NNS) [47] (Sect. 5.6).

4.6.2 Balanced Identification Index (BII)

Balanced Accuracy (BAcc) has been defined (Sect. 2.3.6) as:

$$BAcc = (Sens + Spec)/2$$

Balanced Inaccuracy (BInacc) is its complement:

$$BInacc = 1 - BAcc$$
$$= (FNR + FPR)/2$$

Using BAcc and BInacc in place of Acc and Inacc, one may characterise a Balanced Identification Index (BII) [36] as:

$$BII = BAcc - BInacc$$
$$= BAcc - (1 - BAcc)$$
$$= 2 \cdot BAcc - 1$$

However, this formulation contributes no additional information, since:

$$BAcc = (Sens + Spec)/2$$

Hence:

$$BII = 2 \cdot \left[(Sens + Spec)/2\right] - 1$$
$$= Sens + Spec - 1$$

This is the formula for the Youden index (Sect. 4.2), the value of which is immediately available from Sens and Spec.

As shown previously (Sect. 3.2.7), when datasets are well-balanced ($P = P' = 0.5$), $UAcc = 2.BAcc - 1$, and hence is equal to BII at this prevalence.

Worked Example: Balanced Identification Index (BII)

In a screening test accuracy study of MACE [23], at the MACE cut-off of $\leq$ 20/30, Sens $= 0.912$ and Spec $= 0.707$ (Sect. 2.2.1).

Hence the value for BAcc (Sect. 3.2.6) at this MACE cut-off is:

$$
\begin{aligned}
BAcc &= (Sens + Spec)/2 \\
&= (0.912 + 0.707)/2 \\
&= 0.810
\end{aligned}
$$

Therefore, the value for BII is:

$$
\begin{aligned}
BII &= 2.BAcc - 1 \\
&= (2 \times 0.810) - 1 \\
&= 0.619 \\
&= Y
\end{aligned}
$$

4.6.3 Unbiased Identification Index (UII)

Using unbiased accuracy (UAcc) and unbiased inaccuracy (UInacc), as previously defined (Sect. 3.2.7), in place of Acc and Inacc, one may characterise an Unbiased Identification Index (UII) [36] as:

$$
\begin{aligned}
UII &= UAcc - UInacc \\
&= UAcc - (1 - UAcc) \\
&= 2 \cdot UAcc - 1
\end{aligned}
$$

Worked Example: Unbiased Identification Index (UII)

In a screening test accuracy study of MACE [23], at the MACE cut-off of $\leq$ 20/30, UAcc $= 0.378$ and UInacc $= 0.622$ (Sect. 3.2.7).

Hence the value for UII at this MACE cut-off is:

$$UII = 2 \cdot UAcc - 1$$
$$= (2 \times 0.378) - 1$$
$$= -0.244$$

The value of UII is negative, as anticipated for any value of UAcc < 1. Indeed, examining the MACE study dataset across the range of test cut-offs, UII > 1 occurred only at the maximum (cut-off $\leq$ 15/30) [36].

4.7 Net Reclassification Improvement (NRI)

Net reclassification improvement or net reclassification index (NRI) may be used to quantify test performance. NRI expresses the change in the proportion of correct classification based on an investigation that has been added to the existing diagnostic information [51]. Most simply, this may be calculated as the difference between prior (pre-test) probability of diagnosis, or prevalence, P (Sect. 1.3.2), and posterior probability or test accuracy, Acc (Sect. 3.2.4) [55]:

$$NRI = \text{posterior probability} - \text{pre-test probability}$$
$$= \text{Accuracy} - \text{Prevalence}$$
$$= Acc - P$$

NRI is claimed to be intuitive and easy to use [55]. Evidently, a highly accurate test may be associated with small NRI if P is high, and a low accuracy test may be associated with large NRI if P is low.

In literal notation (Fig. 1.1):

$$NRI = [(TP + TN)/(TP + FP + FN + TN)] - [(TP + FN)/N]$$
$$= [(TP + TN)/N] - [(TP + FN)/N]$$
$$= (TN - FN)/N$$

In algebraic notation (Fig. 1.2):

$$NRI = [(a + d)/(a + b + c + d)] - [(a + c)/N]$$
$$= [(a + d)/N] - [(a + c)/N]$$
$$= (d - c)/N$$

In terms of marginal totals:

$$NRI = r/N - p/N$$
$$= R - P$$

Worked Example: Net Reclassification Improvement (NRI)

In a screening test accuracy study of MACE [23], in a cohort of 755 consecutive patients the prevalence of dementia was $114/755 = 0.151$ (Sect. 1.3.2). At the MACE cut-off giving maximal Youden index for dementia diagnosis, $\leq 20/30$, $TP = 104$, $FN = 10$, $FP = 188$, and $TN = 453$, Acc was 0.738 (Sect. 3.2.4).

Hence the value for NRI at this cut-off is:

$$\begin{aligned} NRI &= Acc - P \\ &= 0.738 - 0.151 \\ &= 0.587 \end{aligned}$$

or

$$\begin{aligned} NRI &= (TN - FN)/N \\ &= (453 - 10)/755 \\ &= 0.587 \end{aligned}$$

NRI might also be characterized in terms of balanced accuracy (Sect. 3.2.6) and unbiased accuracy (Sect. 3.2.7), as balanced NRI (BNRI) and unbiased NRI (UNRI) respectively:

$$BNRI = BAcc - P$$
$$UNRI = UAcc - P$$

Worked Example: Balanced NRI (BNRI) and Unbiased NRI (UNRI)

In a screening test accuracy study of MACE [23], in a cohort of 755 consecutive patients with a prevalence of dementia $P = 0.151$ (Sect. 1.3.2), at the MACE cut-off of $\leq 20/30$, $BAcc = 0.810$ (Sect. 3.2.6) and $UAcc = 0.378$ (Sect. 3.2.7).

Hence the values for BNRI and UNRI at this MACE cut-off are:

$$\begin{aligned} BNRI &= BAcc - P \\ &= 0.810 - 0.151 \\ &= 0.659 \end{aligned}$$

$$\begin{aligned} UNRI &= UAcc - P \\ &= 0.378 - 0.151 \\ &= 0.227 \end{aligned}$$

Hence, as anticipated, since BAcc > Acc > UAcc (Sects. 3.2.5, 3.2.6, 3.2.7), BNRI > NRI > UNRI.

Other usages of "net reclassification improvement" based on reclassification tables may be used ([18], p.199–201).

4.8 Methods to Combine Sens and PPV

4.8.1 Critical Success Index (CSI) or Threat Score (TS)

This parameter, variously known as the critical success index (CSI) [11, 56], or threat score (TS) [49], or ratio of verification [13], had its origin in the context of weather forecasting, specifically tornado predictions [13]. (It was in response to this paper that Peirce proposed measures called the "science of the method," equivalent to the Youden index (Sect. 4.2), and the "utility of the method" (Sect. 3.2.4) [50]). It is equivalent to a measure described by Jaccard, known as the Jaccard index or similarity coefficient, sometimes denoted J. Published in English in 1912 [21], some authors [14] cite a 1908 paper [20] and others [54] a 1901 paper [19] as the forerunner of the English translation. In set theory the Jaccard similarity coefficient represents union over intersection, which was also proposed independently by Tanimoto in 1958 [60], a measure known as the Tanimoto index.

The preferred term here is the critical success index (CSI). In terms of the standard outcomes of signal detection theory, it has been defined as the ratio of hits to the sum of hits, false alarms, and misses. This might also be characterised (Sect. 1.2) as the ratio of true positives to the sum of true positives, false positives, and false negatives.

In literal notation:

$$CSI = TP/(TP + FN + FP)$$

In algebraic notation:

$$CSI = a/(a + b + c)$$

CSI may also be expressed in terms of Sens and PPV:

$$CSI = 1/[(1/PPV) + (1/\,Sens) - 1]$$

CSI ranges from 0 to 1 (perfect forecast).

Worked Example: Critical Success Index (CSI)

In a screening test accuracy study of MACE [23], the MACE cut-off giving maximal Youden index for dementia diagnosis was $\leq 20/30$, where TP $= 104$, FN $= 10$, and FP $= 188$.

Hence the value for CSI is:

$$CSI = TP/(TP + FN + FP)$$
$$= 104/(104 + 10 + 188)$$
$$= 0.344$$

In the screening test accuracy study of MACE, the values for Sens and PPV at cut-off $\leq 20/30$ were 0.912 (Sect. 2.2.1) and 0.356 (Sect. 2.3.1) respectively. Hence the value for CSI calculated using these measures is:

$$CSI = 1/[(1/PPV) + (1/Sens) - 1]$$
$$= 1/[(1/0.356) + (1/0.912) - 1]$$
$$= 1/2.905$$
$$= 0.344$$

Ignoring TN ($= 453$), the calculated CSI suggests MACE is a poor forecaster of the diagnosis of dementia at this cut-off.

Obviously, CSI ignores true negatives (TN, or d), or correct "non-events" as is implicit within its definition:

$$CSI = TP/(N - TN)$$

Part of the rationale for the initial development of the critical success index was to avoid over-inflation of test measures as a consequence of very large numbers of true negatives [13] (i.e. class skew or imbalance), for example measures such as specificity ($= d/(b + d)$) and correct classification accuracy ($= (a + d)/N$).

CSI is dependent on P (see [62]) and Q, and may be expressed in terms of P, Q, and either Sens or PPV. Since (from Sect. 2.3.4) PPV $=$ Sens.P/Q, then:

$$CSI = 1/[(Q/Sens \cdot P) + (1/Sens) - 1]$$
$$= Sens/[1 + Q/P - Sens]$$
$$= Sens/(Q/P) + FNR$$
$$= Sens \cdot P/(Q + P) - Sens \cdot P$$
$$= 1/[(Q + P)/Sens \cdot P] - 1$$

Likewise, since Sens $=$ PPV.Q/P (Sect. 2.3.4), then:

$$CSI = 1/[(1/PPV) + (P/PPV \cdot Q) - 1]$$
$$= PPV/[1 + P/Q - PPV]$$
$$= PPV/(P/Q) + FDR$$
$$= PPV \cdot Q/(Q + P) - PPV \cdot Q$$
$$= 1/[(Q + P)/PPV \cdot Q] - 1$$

Worked Example: Critical Success Index (CSI)

In a screening test accuracy study of MACE [23], at the MACE cut-off giving maximal Youden index for dementia diagnosis ($\leq$20/30), Sens $= 0.912$ (Sect. 2.2.1), P $= 0.151$ and Q $= 0.387$ (Sect. 1.3.2).

Hence the value for CSI is:

$$CSI = 1/[(Q + P)/Sens \cdot P] - 1$$
$$= 1/[0.538/(0.912 \times 0.151)] - 1$$
$$= 0.344$$

In the screening test accuracy study of MACE, the value for PPV at cut-off $\leq$ 20/30 was 0.356 (Sect. 2.3.1).

Hence the value for CSI is:

$$CSI = 1/[(Q + P)/PPV.Q] - 1$$
$$= 1/[0.538/(0.356 \times 0.387)] - 1$$
$$= 0.344$$

Confidence intervals for CSI may be calculated. Clearly the log method (Sects. 2.3.5 and 5.11) is not appropriate here since true negatives are eschewed in the calculation of CSI. Hence the simple method, as used as for sensitivity, specificity, and predictive values, $p \pm 1.96\sqrt{p.(1-p)/n}$, may be applied (Sect. 1.7), using as the denominator n the sum of (TP + FP + FN). In other words, CSI is treated as a proportion and a non-exact binomial method may be used to calculate confidence intervals.

Worked Example: Confidence Intervals for CSI

In a screening test accuracy study of MACE [23], the MACE cut-off giving maximal Youden index for dementia diagnosis was $\leq$20/30, where TP $= 104$, FN $= 10$, and FP $= 188$. The calculated value of CSI was 0.344.

Hence the 95% confidence intervals (95% CI) for CSI are:

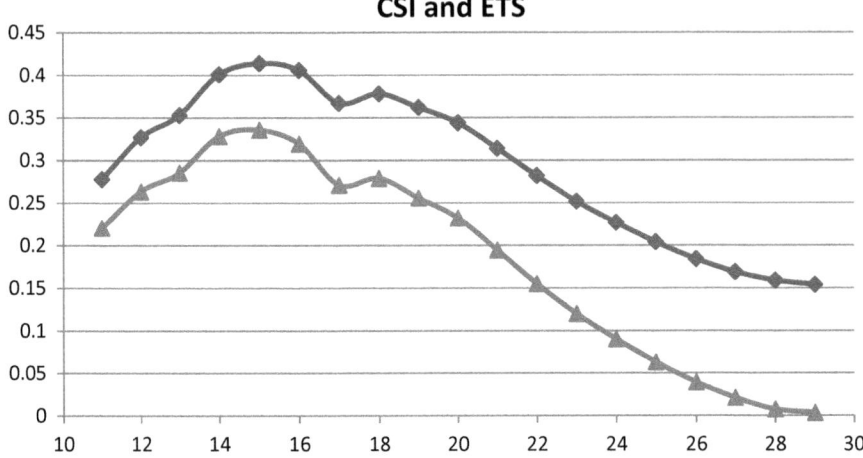

Fig. 4.7 Plot of CSI (diamonds) and ETS (triangles) on y-axis versus MACE cut-off (x axis) [34]

$$95\%CI = 1.96\sqrt{p.(1-p)/n}$$
$$= 0.344 + / - 1.96\sqrt{0.344 \cdot (1 - 0.344)/302}$$
$$= 0.344 + / - 0.0536$$

$$CSI = 0.344(95\%CI = 0.291 - 0.398)$$

CSI values vary with test cut-off or Q (Fig. 4.7), with maximum identical to HMYPSI and MCC in this dataset (Table 7.2). A rescaled quality CSI, QCSI, may be calculated (Sect. 6.5.6).

Jaccard also proposed a dissimilarity coefficient or distance. In the terminology used here, this is given by $(1-CSI)$ and is ideally 0:

In literal notation:

$$1 - CSI = (FP + FN)/(TP + FN + FP)$$
$$= (FP + FN)/(N - TN)$$

Worked Example: Jaccard Distance

In a screening test accuracy study of MACE [23], the MACE cut-off giving maximal Youden index for dementia diagnosis was $\leq 20/30$, where TP $= 104$, FN $= 10$, and FP $= 188$.

Hence the value for Jaccard distance is:

$$1 - CSI = (FP + FN)/(TP + FN + FP)$$
$$= (188 + 10)/(104 + 10 + 188)$$
$$= 198/302$$
$$= 0.656$$

4.8.2 *Equitable Threat Score (ETS) or Gilbert Skill Score*

CSI is not unbiased, since $CSI = TP/(N-TN) = a/(N-d)$, and hence gives lower scores for rarer events. To offset this, a related score may be used to account for hits expected by chance. This is the equitable threat score (ETS) [12], also known as the Gilbert skill score [56]:

$$ETS = a - a_r/(a + b + c - a_r)$$

where

a_r = (total forecasts of event).(total observations of event)/sample size

In literal notation:

$$a_r = (TP + FP)(TP + FN)/N$$

In algebraic notation:

$$a_r = (a + b) \cdot (a + c)/N$$

In terms of marginal totals:

$$a_r = q \cdot p/N$$

Substituting, in literal notation:

$$ETS = [TP - (TP + FP).(TP + FN)/N]/\left[TP + FN + FP - (TP + FP).(TP + FN)/N\right]$$

In algebraic notation:

$$ETS = [a - (a + b) \cdot (a + c)/N]/[a + b + c - (a + b) \cdot (a + c)/N]$$

In terms of marginal totals:

$$ETS = (a - q \cdot p/N)/(a + b + c - q \cdot p/N)$$

This correction for chance is analogous to that used in the kappa statistic (Sect. 8.4.2). ETS values range from $-1/3$ to 1, and are lower than CSI values.

Worked Example: Equitable Threat Score (ETS)

In a screening test accuracy study of MACE [23], the MACE cut-off giving maximal Youden index for dementia diagnosis was $\leq 20/30$, where $TP = 104$, $FN = 10$, and $FP = 188$.

Hence the value for a_r is:

$$a_r = (TP + FP) \cdot (TP + FN)/N$$
$$= (104 + 188) \cdot (104 + 10)/755$$
$$= 44.09$$

Substituting, the value for ETS is:

$$ETS = TP - a_r/(TP + FN + FP) - a_r$$
$$= (104 - 44.09)/(104 + 10 + 188) - 44.09$$
$$= 0.232$$

The calculated ETS suggests MACE is a poor forecaster of diagnosis of dementia at this cut-off, as for CSI.

CSI and ETS values have only recently been used in the characterisation of screening and diagnostic test accuracy studies [34, 37, 42, 45], but as the examples show they are easy to calculate, hence the case for their wider adoption has been advocated [43].

4.8.3   F Measure (F) or F1 Score (Dice Co-efficient)

The F measure (F) or F1 score [53, 54] is defined as the harmonic mean of precision or positive predictive value (PPV; Sect. 2.3.1) and sensitivity or recall (Sect. 2.2.1). This corresponds to the coefficient described by Dice in 1948 [10], hence sometimes denoted D, and independently by Sørensen [59].

In literal notation:

$$F = 2 \cdot TP/(2 \cdot TP + FP + FN)$$

In algebraic notation:

$$F = 2a/(2a + b + c)$$

F may also be expressed in terms of Sens and PPV:

$$F = 2 \cdot PPV \cdot Sens/(PPV + Sens)$$
$$= 2/[1/Sens + 1/PPV]$$

F has range of 0 to 1, where 1 is perfect precision and recall [53].

Worked Example: F Measure (F)

In a screening test accuracy study of the MACE (N = 755) [23], at the cut-off giving maximal Youden index for dementia diagnosis, ≤20/30, TP = 104, FN = 10, and FP = 188.

Hence the value for F is:

$$F = 2 \cdot TP/(2 \cdot TP + FP + FN)$$
$$= (2 \times 104)/([2 \times 104] + 188 + 10)$$
$$= 208/406$$
$$= 0.512$$

This may also be calculated using values of Sens = 0.912 (Sect. 2.2.1) and PPV = 0.356 (Sect. 2.3.1):

$$F = 2 \cdot PPV \cdot Sens/(PPV + Sens)$$
$$= 2 \times 0.356 \times 0.912/(0.356 + 0.912)$$
$$= 0.649/1.268$$
$$= 0.512$$

F is dependent on P and Q, may be expressed in terms of P, Q, and either Sens or PPV [54]:

$$F = 2 \cdot Sens \cdot P/(Q + P)$$
$$= 2 \cdot PPV \cdot Q/(Q + P)$$

Worked Example: F Measure (F)

In a screening test accuracy study of MACE [23], at the MACE cut-off giving maximal Youden index for dementia diagnosis ($\leq$20/30), Sens $= 0.912$ (Sect. 2.2.1), P $= 0.151$ and Q $= 0.387$ (Sect. 1.3.2).

Hence the value for F is:

$$F = 2 \cdot \text{Sens} \cdot P/(Q + P)$$
$$= (2 \times 0.356 \times 0.387)/(0.538)$$
$$= 0.512$$

In the screening test accuracy study of MACE, the value for PPV at cut-off $\leq$20/30 was 0.356 (Sect. 2.3.1). Hence:

$$F = 2 \cdot \text{Sens} \cdot P/(Q + P)$$
$$= (2 \times 0.912 \times 0.151)/(0.538)$$
$$= 0.512$$

F measure ignores true negatives (TN or d), or correct "non-events", as does CSI (Sect. 4.8.1). There is a monotonic relation between the two measures [22], such that:

$$F = 2CSI/(1 + CSI)$$

Worked Examples: Relation of F to CSI

Since F is related to CSI by the equation $F = 2CSI/(1 + CSI)$, if CSI $= 0.344$, then we would expect that:

$$F = 2CSI/(1 + CSI)$$
$$= 2 \times 0.344/(1 + 0.344)$$
$$= 0.512$$
$$\text{QED}$$

Hence, when comparing different tests, the ranking is the same for F and CSI [22, 34] and the plot of F measure values against test cut-off [27] has the same maximum as for CSI and ETS (Fig. 4.7). As for CSI, a case for using F for test evaluation when there are large numbers of TN has been presented [37].

F measure has been calculated for several cognitive screening instruments [26] and varies with test cut-off or Q [27]. A rescaled quality F measure, QF, may be

Table 4.4 Values of PPV (from Table 3.3), Sens (from Table 3.1), and F for dementia diagnosis at fixed MACE cut-off of ≤20/30 at various prevalence levels

P, P′	PPV	Sens	F
0.1, 0.9	0.257	0.914	0.401
0.2, 0.8	0.437	0.908	0.590
0.3, 0.7	0.571	0.896	0.697
0.4, 0.6	0.675	0.884	0.765
0.5, 0.5	0.757	0.865	0.807
0.6, 0.4	0.824	0.840	0.832
0.7, 0.3	0.879	0.803	0.839
0.8, 0.2	0.926	0.746	0.826
0.9, 0.1	0.966	0.640	0.770

calculated (Sect. 6.5.6). F measure also varies with prevalence: for the MACE study (Table 4.4; Fig. 4.8) the optimum value of F is at P = 0.7 (cf. Y and PSI). CSI would be anticipated to vary with P in the same manner.

F measure is a scalar value based on information from both columns of the 2 × 2 table (cf. Sens and Spec), hence varies with prevalence, P (Sect. 2.3.2), as well as with the level of the test, Q, and hence with test cut-off [27] and is also sensitive to class imbalance. Nevertheless, it has been advocated as a measure of agreement, using the nomenclature "proportion of specific positive agreement" (PA) [9], in preference to Cohen's kappa statistic (Sect. 8.4.2). Although the kappa statistic is often characterised as a measure of agreement, it is a relative measure and hence may be characterised as a measure of reliability. In this context, de Vet et al. [9] also characterised a "proportion of specific negative agreement" (NA):

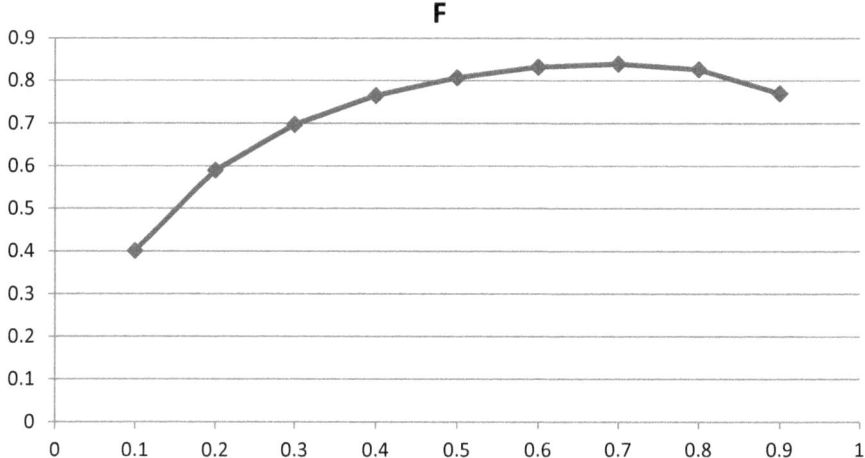

Fig. 4.8 Plot of F (y axis) for dementia diagnosis at fixed Q (MACE cut-off ≤20/30) versus prevalence P (x axis)

$$NA = 2 \cdot TN/(2TN + FP + FN)$$
$$= 2d/(2d + b + c)$$

Evidently this is equivalent to the harmonic mean of Spec and NPV:

$$NA = 2 \cdot NPV \cdot Spec/(NPV + Spec)$$
$$= 2/(1/Spec + 1/NPV)$$

Thus, NA ignores true positives (TP or a), or "hits". It has a range of 0–1, where 1 is perfect NPV and specificity.

It is argued that these measures of specific agreement, PA and NA, facilitate clinical decision making in a way that relative measures such as Cohen's kappa do not [9].

Worked Example: Proportion of Specific Negative Agreement (NA)

In a screening test accuracy study of the MACE (N = 755) [23], at the cut-off giving maximal Youden index for dementia diagnosis, ≤20/30, FN = 10, FP = 188, and TN = 453.

Hence the value for NA is:

$$NA = 2 \cdot TN/(2 \cdot TN + FP + FN)$$
$$= (2 \times 453)/([2 \times 453] + 188 + 10]$$
$$= 906/1104$$
$$= 0.821$$

This may also be calculated using values of Spec = 0.707 (Sect. 2.2.1) and NPV = 0.978 (Sect. 2.3.1):

$$NA = 2 \cdot NPV \cdot Spec/(NPV + Spec)$$
$$= 2 \times 0.978 \times 0.707/(0.978 + 0.707)$$
$$= 1.383/1.685$$
$$= 0.821$$

4.8.4   F*: CSI by Another Name

The appropriateness of combining two aspects of performance as conceptually distinct as PPV (patient-oriented) and Sens (test-oriented) may be questioned, likewise whether their harmonic mean, the F measure, is the best way to combine them

[54]. Accordingly, Hand et al. [14] have described a simple transformation of the F measure which they call "F*", such that:

$$F^* = F/(2 - F)$$
$$= TP/(N - TN)$$
$$= PPV \times Sens/PPV + Sens - (PPV \times Sens)$$

As will be seen from the worked example, F* may be shown to equate to CSI using several elementary mathematical methods, specifically: from the value of F; from the base data of the cells of the 2 × 2 matrix; from the measures of Sens and PPV; and from Sens, P, PPV, and Q [44].

Worked Example: F*

In a screening test accuracy study of the MACE (N = 755) [23], at the cut-off giving maximal Youden index for dementia diagnosis, ≤20/30, F = 0.512, TP = 104, TN = 453, Sens = 0.912, PPV = 0.356, P = 0.151, and Q = 0.387. Hence, using the definition of Hand et al. [14], the value for F* is:

$$F^* = F/(2 - F)$$
$$= 0.512/(2 - 0.512)$$
$$= 0.344$$

Or, expressed using the base data from the 2 × 2 matrix:

$$F^* = TP/(N - TN)$$
$$= 104/(755 - 453)$$
$$= 0.344$$

Or, expressed using values of PPV and Sens:

$$F^* = PPV \times Sens/PPV + Sens - (PPV \times Sens)$$
$$= 0.356 \times 0.912/0.356 + 0.912 - (0.356 \times 0.912)$$
$$= 0.344$$

Or, expressed using values of Sens, P, PPV, and Q:

$$F^* = F/(2 - F)$$

$$F = 2 \cdot Sens \cdot P/(Q + P)$$
$$= 2 \cdot PPV \cdot Q/(Q + P)$$

Substituting and rearranging

$$F^* = [2 \cdot \text{Sens} \cdot P/(Q+P)]/(2 - [2 \cdot \text{Sens} \cdot P/(Q+P)]$$
$$= 1/[(Q+P)/\text{Sens} \cdot P) - 1$$
$$= 1/[(0.538)/(0.912 \times 0.151)] - 1$$
$$= 0.344$$

$$F^* = [2 \cdot \text{PPV} \cdot Q/(Q+P)]/(2 - [2 \cdot \text{PPV} \cdot Q/(Q+P)]$$
$$= 1/[(Q+P)/\text{PPV} \cdot Q) - 1$$
$$= 1/[(0.538)/(0.356 \times 0.387)] - 1$$
$$= 0.344$$

Hence: $F^* = \text{CSI} = F/(2-F) = TP/(N-TN) = \text{PPV} \times \text{Sens/PPV} + \text{Sens} - (\text{PPV} \times \text{Sens}) = 1/[(Q+P)/\text{Sens.P}] - 1 = 1/[(Q+P)/\text{PPV.Q}] - 1$.

F^* is thus simply the latest redescription (or convergent evolution) of a measure periodically described in different fields, including Gilbert's "ratio of verification" (1884), the Jaccard similarity coefficient (1901, 1912), the threat score (1949), the Tanimoto index (1958), and the critical success index (1975, 1990) [44].

4.9 Summary Utility Index (SUI) and Summary Disutility Index (SDI)

A "summary utility index" (SUI) has been proposed [24, 28], based on the clinical utility indexes [48] (Sect. 2.4.2), defined as:

$$\text{SUI} = (\text{PCUI} + \text{NCUI})$$
$$= (\text{Sens} \times \text{PPV}) + (\text{Spec} \times \text{NPV})$$

SUI may thus range from 0 to 2, as for the "gain in certainty" [7] or overall correct classification rate [52] measure derived from Sens and Spec (see Sect. 3.2.4). SUI is therefore desirably as close to 2 as possible. It may be qualitatively classified, based on CUI values (Sect. 2.4.2), as: excellent ≥ 1.62, good ≥ 1.28, adequate ≥ 0.98, poor ≥ 0.72, or very poor < 0.72 [24, 28].

In literal notation:

$$\begin{aligned} \text{SUI} &= [\text{TP}/(\text{TP}+\text{FN}) \times \text{TP}/(\text{TP}+\text{FP})] + [[\text{TN}/(\text{FP}+\text{TN}) \times \text{TN}/(\text{FN}+\text{TN})] \\ &= \text{TP}^2/[(\text{TP}+\text{FN})(\text{TP}+\text{FP})] + \text{TN}^2/[(\text{FP}+\text{TN})(\text{FN}+\text{TN})] \\ &= \text{TP}^2/(p \cdot q) + \text{TN}^2/(p' \cdot q') \end{aligned}$$

In algebraic notation:

$$\begin{aligned} \text{SUI} &= [a/(a+c) \times a/(a+b)] + [[d/(b+d) \times d/(c+d)] \\ &= a^2/[(a+c) \cdot (a+b)] + d^2/[(b+d)(c+d)] \end{aligned}$$

and in terms of marginal totals:

$$\text{SUI} = a^2/(p \cdot q) + d^2/(p' \cdot q')$$

Worked Example: Summary Utility Index (SUI)

In a screening test accuracy study of MACE [23], at the MACE cut-off of $\leq 20/30$ for dementia diagnosis TP = 104, FN = 10, FP = 188, and TN = 453.

The values for Sens and Spec (Sect. 2.2.1) are:

$$\text{Sens} = 0.912$$
$$\text{Spec} = 0.707$$

The values for PPV and NPV (Sect. 2.3.1) are:

$$\text{PPV} = 0.356$$
$$\text{NPV} = 0.978$$

Hence the values for PCUI and NCUI (Sect. 2.4.2) are:

$$\begin{aligned} \text{PCUI} &= \text{Sens} \times \text{PPV} \\ &= 0.912 \times 0.356 \\ &= 0.325 \end{aligned}$$

$$\begin{aligned} \text{NCUI} &= \text{Spec} \times \text{NPV} \\ &= 0.707 \times 0.978 \\ &= 0.691 \end{aligned}$$

Hence the value for SUI is:

$$SUI = PCUI \times NCUI$$
$$= 0.325 \times 0.691$$
$$= 1.016$$

This value of SUI is qualitatively classified as adequate.

SUI values have been calculated for many neurological signs and cognitive screening questions and instruments [23, 24, 29–32]. SUI values vary with test cut-off or Q [23], with the same maximum as for other unitary measures such as HMYPSI, MCC, CSI and F measure [27] (Table 7.2). SUI also varies with prevalence ([28], p.163–5). SUI may be rescaled according to the level of the test, Q [25], as QSUI (Sect. 6.5.7).

The reciprocal (multiplicative inverse) of SUI has been termed the number needed for screening utility (NNSU; Sect. 5.14) [24, 28].

A "summary disutility index" (SDI) may also be proposed (first described as such in [33], p.93–4) based on the clinical disutility indexes (Sect. 2.4.3), defined as:

$$SDI = (PCDI + NCDI)$$
$$= (FNR \times FDR) + (FPR \times FRR)$$

SDI may thus range from 0 to 2, as for SUI, and is desirably as close to 0 as possible. It may be qualitatively classified, based on CDI values (Sect. 2.4.3), as: very poor ≥ 1.62, poor ≥ 1.28, adequate ≥ 0.98, good ≥ 0.72, or excellent < 0.72 (i.e. higher score worse).

Worked Example: Summary Disutility Index (SDI)

In a screening test accuracy study of MACE [23], at the MACE cut-off of $\leq 20/30$ for dementia diagnosis TP = 104, FN = 10, FP = 188, and TN = 453.

The values for FNR and FPR (Sect. 2.2.3) are:

$$FNR = 0.088$$
$$FPR = 0.293$$

The values for FDR and FRR (Sect. 2.3.3) are:

$$FDR = 0.644$$
$$FRR = 0.022$$

Hence the values for PCDI and NCDI (Sect. 2.4.2) are:

$$PCDI = FNR \times FDR$$
$$= 0.088 \times 0.644$$
$$= 0.057$$

$$NCDI = FPR \times FRR$$
$$= 0.293 \times 0.022$$
$$= 0.006$$

Hence the value for SDI is:

$$SDI = PCDI \times NCDI$$
$$= 0.057 \times 0.006$$
$$= 0.063$$

This value of SDI is qualitatively classified as excellent.

As for SUI, SDI may be rescaled according to the level of the test, Q (Sect. 6.5.7). The reciprocal (multiplicative inverse) of SDI has been termed the number needed for screening disutility (NNDU; Sect. 5.15).

4.10 "Diagnostic Yield"

Another unitary construct sometimes encountered in test evaluation is "yield" or "diagnostic yield" or "detection rate". This may be defined as the likelihood that a test provides positive findings, or the information needed to establish a diagnosis, or the proportion of tests producing a specific diagnosis (e.g.[8]). Values for diagnostic yield range from 0 to 1, and are often expressed as percentages.

It seems evident to me that there is ambiguity in the definition of "diagnostic yield". It might mean only the proportion of true positives (= TP/N). If the study simply examines a case series, then N might in fact be equal to p, and hence yield = TP/p (Sect. 2.2.1). Lim et al. calculated the "diagnostic yield" of MR imaging in transient global amnesia (TGA) as the ratio of the number of patients with small hyperintense MR-DWI lesions suggestive of TGA to the total number of patients with TGA [39]. Previously ([38], p.85), I thought that this usage equated to test sensitivity (i.e. ratio of true positives to sum of true positives and false negatives = TP/p), but on re-reading the paper I now think it might simply be TP/N (although this might equate to TP/p if no non-TGA cases were included). In a population or case–control study, "yield" might refer to all positive tests, both true and false (= (TP + FP)/N). As discussed previously (Sect. 1.3.2), this measure is also known as the positive sign rate, or Q, or bias. If TP >>> FP, then diagnostic yield would approximate to TP/N.

The "diagnostic yield" terminology would thus seem to be at risk of underspecification. If used to mean TP/p, it may overestimate test utility, as this ignores FP, and a priori it seems unlikely that any test can entirely avoid FP instances. If used to mean TP/N, then careful specification of "N" is required to understand whether FN and FP case are included in N. Use of relative TP and FP fractions [8] may perhaps go some way to circumvent the ambiguity inherent in the term "diagnostic yield".

Worked Example: "Diagnostic Yield"

In a screening test accuracy study of the MACE (N = 755) [23], at the MACE cut-off of ≤20/30 for dementia diagnosis TP = 104 and FP = 188.
If "diagnostic yield" = TP/N, then:

$$TP/N = 104/755$$
$$= 0.138$$

If "diagnostic yield" = (TP + FP)/N, then:

$$(TP + FP)/N = (104 + 188)/755$$
$$= 0.387$$
$$= Q$$

Since in this instance FP > TP, the outcome of the different calculations of "diagnostic yield" is substantial.
If "diagnostic yield" = TP/p, then:

$$TP/N = 104/114$$
$$= 0.912$$
$$= Sens$$

With the wide variety of other parameters available from the 2 × 2 contingency table to characterise test outcome, it is the view of this author that "diagnostic yield", however defined, has little to recommend it in comparison to other measures. Indeed, some studies reporting "diagnostic yield" appear to use the term in a generic way to encompass various parameters including sensitivity, specificity, predictive values, and area under the ROC curve.

References

1. Baker SG, Kraemer BS. Peirce, Youden, and receiver operating characteristic curves. Am Stat. 2007;61:343–6.
2. Boughorbel S, Jarray F, El-Anbari M. Optimal classifier for imbalanced data using Matthews Correlation Coefficient metric. PLoS ONE. 2017;12(6): e0177678.
3. Brenner H, Gefeller O. Variation of sensitivity, specificity, likelihood ratios and predictive values with disease prevalence. Stat Med. 1997;16:981–91.
4. Chicco D. Ten quick tips for machine learning in computational biology. BioData Min. 2017;10:35.
5. Chicco D, Jurman G. The advantages of the Matthews correlation coefficient (MCC) over F1 score and accuracy in binary classification evaluation. BMC Genomics. 2020;21:6.
6. Chicco D, Tötsch N, Jurman G. The Matthews correlation coefficient (MCC) is more reliable than balanced accuracy, bookmaker informedness, and markedness in two-class confusion matrix evaluation. BioData Mining. 2021;14:13.
7. Connell FA, Koepsell TD. Measures of gain in certainty from a diagnostic test. Am J Epidemiol. 1985;121:744–53.
8. de Haan MC, Nio CY, Thomeer M, et al. Comparing the diagnostic yields of technologists and radiologists in an invitational colorectal cancer screening program performed with CT colonography. Radiology. 2012;264:771–8.
9. De Vet HCW, Mokkink LB, Terwee CB, Hoekstra OS, Knol DL. Clinicians are right not to like Cohen's κ. BMJ. 2013;346: f2515.
10. Dice LR. Measures of the amount of ecological association between species. Ecology. 1945;26:297–302.
11. Donaldson RJ, Dyer RM, Kraus MJ. An objective evaluator of techniques for predicting severe weather events. Preprints, 9th Conference on Severe Local Storms. Norman, Oklahoma, 1975: 312–326.
12. Doswell CA III, Davies-Jones R, Keller DL. On summary measures of skill in rare event forecasting based on contingency tables. Weather Forecast. 1990;5:576–85.
13. Gilbert GK. Finley's tornado predictions. Am Meteorol J. 1884;1:166–72.
14. Hand DJ, Christen P, Kirielle N. F*: an interpretable transformation of the F measure. Mach Learn. 2021;110:451–6.
15. Heston TF. Standardized predictive values. J Magn Reson Imaging. 2014;39:1338.
16. Hilden J, Glasziou P. Regret graphs, diagnostic uncertainty and Youden's index. Stat Med. 1996;15:969–86.
17. Hsieh S, McGrory S, Leslie F, Dawson K, Ahmed S, Butler CR, et al. The Mini-Addenbrooke's Cognitive Examination: a new assessment tool for dementia. Dement Geriatr Cogn Disord. 2015;39:1–11.
18. Hunink MGM, Weinstein MC, Wittenberg E, Drummond MF, Pliskin JS, Wong JB, et al. Decision making in health and medicine. Integrating evidence and values. 2nd edn. Cambridge: Cambridge University Press; 2014.
19. Jaccard P. Étude comparative de la distribution florale dans une portion des Alpes et des Jura. Bulletin de la Société Vaudoise des Sciences Naturelles. 1901;37:547–79.
20. Jaccard P. Nouvelles recherches sur la distribution florale. Bulletin de la Société Vaudoise des Sciences Naturelles. 1908;44:223–70.
21. Jaccard P. The distribution of the flora in the alpine zone. New Phytol. 1912;11:37–50.
22. Jolliffe IT. The Dice co-efficient: a neglected verification performance measure for deterministic forecasts of binary events. Meteorol Appl. 2016;23:89–90.
23. Larner AJ. MACE for diagnosis of dementia and MCI: examining cut-offs and predictive values. Diagnostics (Basel). 2019;9:E51.
24. Larner AJ. New unitary metrics for dementia test accuracy studies. Prog Neurol Psychiatry. 2019;23(3):21–5.
25. Larner AJ. Applying Kraemer's Q (positive sign rate): some implications for diagnostic test accuracy study results. Dement Geriatr Cogn Dis Extra. 2019;9:389–96.

26. Larner AJ. What is test accuracy? Comparing unitary accuracy metrics for cognitive screening instruments. Neurodegener Dis Manag. 2019;9:277–81.
27. Larner AJ. Defining "optimal" test cut-off using global test metrics: evidence from a cognitive screening instrument. Neurodegener Dis Manag. 2020;10:223–30.
28. Larner AJ. Manual of screeners for dementia: pragmatic test accuracy studies. London: Springer; 2020.
29. Larner AJ. Mini-Addenbrooke's Cognitive Examination (MACE): a useful cognitive screening instrument in older people? Can Geriatr J. 2020;23:199–204.
30. Larner AJ. Mini-Cog versus Codex (cognitive disorders examination): is there a difference? Dement Neuropsychol. 2020;14:128–33.
31. Larner AJ. Screening for dementia: Q* index as a global measure of test accuracy revisited. medRxiv. 2020. https://doi.org/10.1101/2020.04.01.20050567
32. Larner AJ. The "attended alone" and "attended with" signs in the assessment of cognitive impairment: a revalidation. Postgrad Med. 2020;132:595–600.
33. Larner AJ. The 2 × 2 matrix. Contingency, confusion and the metrics of binary classification. London: Springer; 2021.
34. Larner AJ. Assessing cognitive screening instruments with the critical success index. Prog Neurol Psychiatry. 2021;25(3):33–7.
35. Larner AJ. Accuracy of cognitive screening instruments reconsidered: overall, balanced, or unbiased accuracy? Neurodegener Dis Manag. 2022;12:67–76.
36. Larner AJ. Evaluating binary classifiers: extending the efficiency index. Neurodegener Dis Manag. 2022;12:185–94.
37. Larner AJ. Intracranial bruit: Charles Warlow's challenge revisited. Pract Neurol. 2022;22:79–81.
38. Larner AJ. Transient global amnesia. From patient encounter to clinical neuroscience. 2nd edn. London: Springer; 2022.
39. Lim SJ, Kim M, Suh CH, Kim SY, Shim WH, Kim SJ. Diagnostic yield of diffusion-weighted brain magnetic resonance imaging in patients with transient global amnesia: a systematic review and meta-analysis. Korean J Radiol. 2021;22:1680–9.
40. Linn S, Grunau PD. New patient-oriented summary measure of net total gain in certainty for dichotomous diagnostic tests. Epidemiol Perspect Innov. 2006;3:11.
41. Matthews BW. Comparison of the predicted and observed secondary structure of T4 phage lysozyme. Biochem Biophys Acta. 1975;405:442–51.
42. Mbizvo GK, Larner AJ. Isolated headache is not a reliable indicator for brain cancer. Clin Med. 2022;22:92–3.
43. Mbizvo GK, Larner AJ. Re: Realistic expectations are key to realising the benefits of polygenic scores. https://www.bmj.com/content/380/bmj-2022-073149/rapid-responses (Published 11 March 2023)
44. Mbizvo GK, Larner AJ. F*, an interpretable transformation of the F measure, equates to the critical success index. *Preprints.org* 2023, 2023090556. https://doi.org/10.20944/preprints202309.0556.v1
45. Mbizvo GK, Bennett KH, Simpson CR, Duncan SE, Chin RFM, Larner AJ. Using Critical Success Index or Gilbert Skill Score as composite measures of positive predictive value and sensitivity in diagnostic accuracy studies: weather forecasting informing epilepsy research. Epilepsia. 2023;64:1466–8.
46. Mendez MF. The mental status examination handbook. Philadelphia: Elsevier; 2022.
47. Mitchell AJ. Index test. In: Kattan MW, editor. Encyclopedia of medical decision making. Los Angeles: Sage; 2009. p. 613–7.
48. Mitchell AJ. Sensitivity × PPV is a recognized test called the clinical utility index (CUI+). Eur J Epidemiol. 2011;26:251–2.
49. Palmer WC, Allen RA. Note on the accuracy of forecasts concerning the rain problem. Washington, DC: U.S. Weather Bureau manuscript; 1949.
50. Peirce CS. The numerical measure of the success of predictions. Science. 1884;4:453–4.

51. Pencina MJ, D'Agostino RB Sr, D'Agostino RB Jr, Vasan RS. Evaluating the added predictive ability of a new marker: from area under the ROC curve to reclassification and beyond. Stat Med. 2008;27:157–72.
52. Perkins NJ, Schisterman EF. The inconsistency of "optimal" cutpoints obtained using two criteria based on the receiver operating characteristic curve. Am J Epidemiol. 2006;163:670–5.
53. Powers DMW. Evaluation: from precision, recall and F-measure to ROC, informedness, markedness and correlation. J Machine Learning Technologies. 2011;2:37–63.
54. Powers DMW. What the F measure doesn't measure … Features, flaws, fallacies and fixes. arXiv. 2015. 1503.06410.2015.
55. Richard E, Schmand BA, Eikelenboom P, Van Gool WA, The Alzheimer's Disease Neuroimaging Initiative. MRI and cerebrospinal fluid biomarkers for predicting progression to Alzheimer's disease in patients with mild cognitive impairment: a diagnostic accuracy study. BMJ Open. 2013;3:e002541.
56. Schaefer JT. The critical success index as an indicator of warning skill. Weather Forecast. 1990;5:570–5.
57. Schisterman EF, Perkins NJ, Liu A, Bondell H. Optimal cut-point and its corresponding Youden index to discriminate individuals using pooled blood samples. Epidemiology. 2005;16:73–81.
58. Smits N. A note on Youden's J and its cost ratio. BMC Med Res Methodol. 2010;10:89.
59. Sørensen T. A method of establishing groups of equal amplitude in plant sociology based on similarity of species and its application to analyses of the vegetation on Danish commons. K Dan Vidensk Sels. 1948;5:1–34.
60. Tanimoto TT. *An elementary mathematical theory of classification and prediction.* Internal IBM Technical Report 17th November 1958. http://dalkescientific.com/tanimoto.pdf
61. Youden WJ. Index for rating diagnostic tests. Cancer. 1950;3:32–5.
62. Mbizvo GK, Larner AJ. On the dependence of the critical success index (CSI) on prevalence. medRxiv. https://doi.org/10.1101/2023.12.03.23299335

Chapter 5
Number Needed (Reciprocal) Measures and Their Combinations as Likelihoods

Contents

5.1 Introduction

This chapter considers reciprocal or "number needed" measures of test outcome which can be derived from the basic 2×2 contingency table, where reciprocal means multiplicative inverse [9, 14]. From these, certain "likelihood" measures may be calculated.

"Number needed" measures originated in the need to describe the outcomes of therapeutic trials in a way that was easily comprehensible for clinicians and their patients. The "number needed to treat" (NNT) is a measure of therapeutic utility [3], equal to the reciprocal of absolute risk reduction, and the "number needed to harm" (NNH) is a measure of the adverse effects of therapeutic interventions [32]. Although quite widely used as an outcome measure in therapeutic trials, NNT is recognised to have limitations, including the unspecified time frame of treatment, and the assumption that benefits are dichotomised rather than partial [30].

Subsequently, adaptations of this "number needed" methodology have been made, for example developing measures such as the "number needed to see" for a specific event or occurrence to be encountered in clinical practice ([8], p.23–4, 39–41). "Number needed" measures have also been developed to summarise the outcomes of diagnostic and screening tests in a manner deemed more intuitive to clinicians and patients than the traditional measures of discrimination such as sensitivity and specificity [24].

When "number needed" measures refer to patients, it is obvious that only positive integer values are clinically meaningful, with absolute ("raw") values being rounded to the next highest integer value for purposes of clinical communication [10].

5.2 Number Needed to Diagnose (NND and NND*)

The reciprocal (multiplicative inverse) of the Youden index, Y (Sect. 4.2), has been defined by Linn and Grunau as the "number needed to diagnose" (NND) [25]. It may be expressed in terms of sensitivity (Sens) and specificity (Spec), and false positive (FPR) and false negative (FNR) rates (Sects. 2.2.1 and 2.2.2):

$$
\begin{aligned}
\text{NND} &= 1/Y \\
&= 1/(\text{Sens} + \text{Spec} - 1) \\
&= 1/\left[\text{Sens} - (1 - \text{Spec})\right] \\
&= 1/(\text{Sens} - \text{FPR}) \\
&= 1/(\text{TPR} - \text{FPR}) \\
&= 1/\left[\text{Spec} - (1 - \text{Sens})\right] \\
&= 1/(\text{Spec} - \text{FNR}) \\
&= 1/(\text{TNR} - \text{FNR}) \\
&= 1/[1 - (\text{FPR} + \text{FNR})]
\end{aligned}
$$

As Y may also be expressed in terms of likelihood ratios (LRs) (Sect. 2.3.5) and correct classification and misclassification rates (Sect. 3.2.4), NND may also be expressed in these terms:

$$
\begin{aligned}
\text{NND} &= 1/[(\text{PLR} - 1) \times (1 - \text{NLR})/(\text{PLR} - \text{NLR})] \\
&= (\text{PLR} - \text{NLR})/[(\text{PLR} - 1) \times (1 - \text{NLR})]
\end{aligned}
$$

$$NND = 1/(\text{ Correct classification rate } - 1)$$
$$= 1/(1 - \text{Misclassification rate})$$

NND may be interpreted as the number of patients who need to be examined (for clinical signs) or tested (with a screening or diagnostic test) in order to detect correctly one person with the disease of interest in a study population of persons with and without the known disease.

In literal notation (see Fig. 1.1):

$$NND = 1/[TP/(TP + FN) + TN/(FP + TN) - 1]$$
$$= 1/\left[TP/p + TN/p' - 1\right]$$

In algebraic notation (see Fig. 1.2):

$$NND = 1/[a/(a + c) + d/(b + d) - 1]$$
$$= (a + c) \cdot (b + d)/ad - bc$$

In error notation (see Fig. 1.5):

$$NND = 1/[1 - (\alpha + \beta)]$$

The range of Y is -1 to $+1$, so 1/Y could theoretically vary from $--1$ to $+1$. However, as the effective range of Y is 0 (no diagnostic value) to 1 (no false positives or false negatives), the anticipated range of 1/Y is ∞ (no diagnostic value) to 1 (no false positives or false negatives).

For diagnostic tests, low values of NND will therefore be desirable.

As the value of Y approaches 0, then NND values become inflated, as for any reciprocal (indeed if $Y = 0$, the division may be characterised as forbidden since it does not yield a unique result and is hence meaningless). This observation has prompted the opinion that NND is not a clinically meaningful number [26]. NND is also (notionally) insensitive to variation in disease prevalence since it depends entirely on Sens and Spec [25]. This shortcoming may be addressed by using the number needed to predict (Sect. 5.3).

Worked Example: Number Needed to Diagnose (NND)

The Mini-Addenbrooke's Cognitive Examination (MACE) [5] was subjected to a screening test accuracy study [10]. At the MACE cut-off of $\leq 20/30$, the values for Sens and Spec (Sect. 2.2.1) were 0.912 and 0.707 respectively.

Hence the value for Y (Sect. 4.2) at this cut-off is:

$$Y = \text{Sens} + \text{Spec} - 1$$

$$= 0.912 + 0.707 - 1$$
$$= 0.619$$

The value for NND is:

$$NND = 1/Y$$
$$= 1/0.619$$
$$= 1.62$$

Referring to patients, NND is rounded up to the next whole integer and is therefore 2.

NND values vary with test cut-off [10]. A rescaled NND, QNND may also be calculated [11] (Sect. 6.6.1).

The NND has certain shortcomings when used in the calculation of likelihood to diagnose or misdiagnose measures (see Sect. 5.6) and for this reason a redefinition of NND as NND* was proposed [19], using Acc rather than Sens and Spec in the denominator, such that:

$$NND^* = 1/Acc$$

In literal notation:

$$NND^* = 1/[(TP + TN)/(TP + FP + FN + TN)]$$
$$= 1/[(TP + TN)/N]$$
$$= N/(TP + TN)$$

In algebraic notation:

$$NND^* = 1/[(a + d)/(a + b + c + d)]$$
$$= 1/[(a + d)/N]$$
$$= N/(a + d)$$

This formulation of NND* is analogous to the definition of the "number needed to misdiagnose" (see Sect. 5.5) [4].

Worked Example: Number Needed to Diagnose (NND*)

In a screening test accuracy study of MACE [10], at the MACE cut-off of $\leq$ 20/30, the value for Acc was 0.738 (Sect. 3.2.5).

Hence the value for NND* is:

$$NND^* = 1/Acc$$
$$= 1/0.738$$
$$= 1.36$$

Alternatively, at this cut-off in the MACE study (N = 755), TP = 104 and TN = 453 (Fig. 2.2).

$$NND^* = N/(TP + TN)$$
$$= 755/(104 + 453)$$
$$= 1.36$$

Referring to patients, NND* is rounded up to the next whole integer and is therefore 2.

NND* has been used in the definition of an Efficiency Index to evaluate binary classifiers (Sect. 5.11) [21].

5.3   Number Needed to Predict (NNP)

The reciprocal (multiplicative inverse) of the predictive summary index, PSI or Ψ (Sect. 4.3), has been defined by Linn and Grunau as the number needed to predict (NNP) [25]. It may be expressed in terms of positive and negative predictive values (PPV, NPV), and false discovery (FDR) and false reassurance (FRR) rates (Sects. 2.3.1 and 2.3.2):

$$NNP = 1/PSI$$
$$= 1/(PPV + NPV - 1)$$
$$= 1/[PPV - (1 - NPV)]$$
$$= 1/(PPV - FRR)$$
$$= 1/[NPV - (1 - PPV)]$$
$$= 1/(NPV - FDR)$$

NNP may be interpreted as the number of patients who need to be examined or tested in the patient population in order to predict correctly the diagnosis of one person.

In literal notation:

$$NNP = 1/[TP/(TP + FP) + TN/(FN + TN) - 1]$$
$$= 1/\left[TP/q + TN/q' - 1\right]$$

In algebraic notation:

$$NNP = 1/[a/(a+b) + d/(c+d) - 1]$$
$$= (a+b).(c+d)/(ad - bc)$$

As the effective range of PSI is 0 (no diagnostic value) to 1 (no false discoveries or false reassurances), the anticipated range of 1/PSI is ∞ (no predictive value) to 1 (no false discoveries or false reassurances). For diagnostic tests, low values of NNP will therefore be desirable. NNP is dependent on disease prevalence and is therefore deemed a better descriptor of diagnostic tests than NND in patient populations with different prevalence of disease [25].

Worked Example: Number Needed To Predict (NNP)

In a screening test accuracy study of MACE [10], at the MACE cut-off of $\leq 20/30$, the values for PPV and NPV (Sect. 2.3.1) were 0.356 and 0.978 respectively.

Hence the value for PSI (Sect. 4.3) at this cut-off is:

$$PSI = PPV + NPV - 1$$
$$= 0.356 + 0.978 - 1$$
$$= 0.334$$

The value for NNP is:

$$NNP = 1/PSI$$
$$= 1/0.334$$
$$= 2.99$$

Referring to patients, NND is rounded up to the next whole integer and is therefore 3.

NNP values vary with test cut-off [10].

5.4 Number Needed to Screen (NNS)

A "number needed to screen" (NNS) measure was first defined for use in public health epidemiology, defined as the number of people that need to be screened for a given duration to prevent one death or adverse event [28].

In terms of screening or diagnostic test accuracy studies, a "number needed to screen" (NNS) measure has been defined as the number of patients who need to be screened in order for one additional correct identification beyond those misidentified [27]. NNS is derived from the identification index (II) (Sect. 4.6.1):

$$\begin{aligned} \text{NNS} &= 1/\text{II} \\ &= 1/[\text{Acc} - (\text{Inacc})] \\ &= 1/[\text{Acc} - (1 - \text{Acc})] \\ &= 1/(2.\text{Acc} - 1) \end{aligned}$$

II ranges from -1 to $+1$ (Sect. 4.6.1), as for Y and PSI. However, whereas negative values are not anticipated with Y and PSI, any value of Acc < 0.5 (i.e. when Inacc > 0.5) will result in a negative value of II, and hence a negative value of NNS. As only positive integer values are clinically meaningful for "number needed" measures when these refer to patients, negative NNS values are clinically meaningless.

In literal notation:

$$\begin{aligned} \text{NNS} &= 1/[2 \cdot (\text{TP} + \text{TN})/(\text{TP} + \text{FP} + \text{FN} + \text{TN}) - 1] \\ &= 1/[2 \cdot (\text{TP} + \text{TN})/\text{N} - 1] \end{aligned}$$

In algebraic notation:

$$\begin{aligned} \text{NNS} &= 1/[2.(a + d)/(a + b + c + d) - 1] \\ &= 1/[2.(a + d)/\text{N} - 1] \end{aligned}$$

Worked Example: Number Needed to Screen (NNS)

In a screening test accuracy study of MACE [10], at the MACE cut-off of $\leq$ 20/30, TP $= 104$, FN $= 10$, FP $= 188$, and TN $= 453$ (Fig. 2.2).

The value for Acc (Sect. 3.2.5) is:

$$\begin{aligned} \text{Acc} &= (\text{TP} + \text{TN})/(\text{TP} + \text{FN} + \text{FP} + \text{TN}) \\ &= (104 + 453)/(104 + 10 + 188 + 453) \\ &= 0.738 \end{aligned}$$

The value for II (Sect. 4.6.1) is:

$$\begin{aligned} \text{II} &= 2 \cdot \text{Acc} - 1 \\ &= (2 \times 0.738) - 1 \\ &= 0.475 \end{aligned}$$

Hence, the value for NNS is:

$$NNS = 1/(2 \cdot Acc - 1)$$
$$= 1/0.475$$
$$= 2.11$$

Referring to patients, NNS is rounded up to the next whole integer and is therefore 3.

NNS varies with test cut-off [10].

It would be possible to calculate NNS values using balanced II (Sect. 4.6.2) or unbiased II (Sect. 4.6.3) rather than II.

5.5 Number Needed to Misdiagnose (NNM)

The reciprocal (multiplicative inverse) of inaccuracy (Sect. 3.2.5) has been defined as the "number needed to misdiagnose" (NNM) [4]:

$$NNM = 1/Inacc$$
$$= 1/(1 - Acc)$$

In literal notation:

$$NNM = 1/[(FP + FN)/(TP + FP + FN + TN)]$$
$$= 1/[(FP + FN)/N]$$
$$= N/(FP + FN)$$

In algebraic notation:

$$NNM = 1/[(b + c)/(a + b + c + d)]$$
$$= 1/[(b + c)/N]$$
$$= N/(b + c)$$

NNM is characterised as a measure of effectiveness, the number of patients who need to be examined or tested in order for one to be misdiagnosed [4]. For diagnostic tests, high values of NNM will therefore be desirable.

Worked Example: Number Needed to Misdiagnose (NNM)

In a screening test accuracy study of MACE [10], at the MACE cut-off of $\leq 20/30$, the values for Acc and Inacc (Sect. 3.2.5) were 0.738 and 0.262 respectively.

Hence the value for NNM at this cut-off is:

$$NNM = 1/Inacc$$
$$= 1(1 - Acc)$$
$$= 1/0.262$$
$$= 3.82$$

Alternatively, at this cut-off in the MACE study ($N = 755$), $FN = 10$ and $FP = 188$ (Fig. 2.2).

$$NNM = N + (FP + FN)$$
$$= 755/(188 + 10)$$
$$= 3.81$$

[The different results relate to rounding errors].

Referring to patients, NNM is rounded up to the next whole integer and is therefore 4.

NNM values vary with test cut-off [10].

5.6 Likelihood to Be Diagnosed or Misdiagnosed (LDM)

Consideration of the numbers needed to diagnose (NND; Sect. 5.2), predict (NNP; Sect. 5.3), and misdiagnose (NNM; Sect. 5.5) prompted the development of measures called the "likelihood to be diagnosed or misdiagnosed" (LDM) and the "likelihood to be predicted or misdiagnosed" (LPM) (Sect. 5.7) [12, 14]. The stimulus for this development came, as for "numbers needed" measures, from therapeutic studies (Sect. 5.1).

The "number needed" measures used to describe therapeutic studies, NNT and NNH (Sect. 5.1), were combined by Citrome and Ketter [2] to produce a "likelihood to be helped or harmed" (LHH) measure to summarise the effects of a therapeutic intervention, where:

$$LHH = NNH/NNT$$

LHH values are ideally as large as possible for therapeutic interventions, since NNH is desirably large and NNT is desirably small. LHH values are reported to help clinicians and patients to evaluate potential risk–benefit trade-offs of treatment [1].

The "likelihood to be diagnosed or misdiagnosed" (LDM) [9, 10, 12, 13] was developed as analogous to LHH but for use in test accuracy studies. Two formulations of LDM were initially proposed:

$$LDM = NNM/NND$$

and:

$$LDM = NNM/NNP$$

The latter might also be termed the "likelihood to be predicted or misdiagnosed" (LPM) to distinguish it from the other formulation; it is considered further in Sect. 5.7.
For LDM = NNM/NND :

$$LDM = [1/(1 - Acc)](1/Y)$$
$$= Y/Inacc$$

In literal notation:

$$LDM = (1/[(FP + FN)/(TP + FP + FN + TN)])/(1/[TP/(TP + FN) + TN/(FP + TN) - 1])$$
$$= (1/[(FP + FN)/(TP + FP + FN + TN)])/(1/[TP/(TP + FN) - FP/(FP + TN)])$$
$$= [TP/(TP + FN) - FP/(FP + TN)]/[(FP + FN)/(TP + FP + FN + TN)]$$

In algebraic notation:

$$LDM = (1/[(b + c)/(a + b + c + d)])/(1/[a/(a + c) + d/(b + d) - 1])$$
$$= (1/[(b + c)/(a + b + c + d)])/(1/[a/(a + c) - b/(b + d)])$$
$$= [a/(a + c) - b/(b + d)]/[(b + c)/(a + b + c + d)]$$

Worked Example: Likelihood To Be Diagnosed Or Misdiagnosed (LDM)

In a screening test accuracy study of MACE [10], at the MACE cut-off of $\leq$ 20/30, the absolute ("raw") values for NND (Sect. 5.2) and NNM (Sect. 5.5) were 1.62 and 3.82 respectively.

Hence the value for LDM at this cut-off is:

$$LDM = NNM/NND$$
$$= 3.82/1.62$$
$$= 2.36$$

LDM may also be calculated from the values of Y (Sect. 4.2) and Inacc (Sect. 3.2.5), as:

$$LDM = Y/Inacc$$
$$= 0.619/0.262$$
$$= 2.36$$

A rescaled, quality form may also be calculated for this variant of LDM [11] (Sect. 6.6.4).

5.7 Likelihood to Be Predicted or Misdiagnosed (LPM)

For the likelihood to be predicted or misdiagnosed:

$$LDM = NNM/NNP$$
$$= [1/(1 - Acc)/(1/PSI)]$$
$$= PSI/Inacc$$

In literal notation:

$$LPM = 1/[(FP + FN)/(TP + FP + FN + TN)]/(1/[TP/(TP + FP) + TN/(FN + TN) - 1])$$
$$= 1/[(FP + FN)/(TP + FP + FN + TN)]/(1/[TP/(TP + FP) - FN/(FN + TN)])$$
$$= [TP/(TP + FP) - FN/(FN + TN)]/[(FP + FN)/(TP + FP + FN + TN)]$$

In algebraic notation:

$$LPM = (1/[(b + c)/(a + b + c + d)])/(1/[a/(a + b) + d/(c + d) - 1])$$
$$= (1/[(b + c)/(a + b + c + d)])/(1/[a/(a + b) - c/(c + d)])$$
$$= [a/(a + b) - c/(c + d)]/[(b + c)/(a + b + c + d)]$$

Worked Example: Likelihood To Be Predicted Or Misdiagnosed (LPM)

In a screening test accuracy study of MACE [10], at the MACE cut-off of $\leq$ 20/30, the absolute ("raw") values for NNP (Sect. 5.3) and NNM (Sect. 5.5) are 2.99, and 3.82 respectively.

Hence the value for LPM at this cut-off is:

$$LPM = NNM/NNP$$
$$= 3.82/2.99$$
$$= 1.28$$

LPM may also be calculated from the values of PSI (Sect. 4.3) and Inacc (Sect. 3.2.5), as:

$$LPM = PSI/Inacc$$
$$= 0.334/0.262$$
$$= 1.27$$

[The different results relate to rounding errors].

A rescaled, quality form of form of LPM may also be calculated (Sect. 6.6.5).

Hence LDM and LPM may be conceptualised as ratios of benefits (correct diagnosis, correct prediction) and harms (misdiagnosis). These may be compared with the net harm to net benefit (H/B) ratio (see Sect. 2.3.6). LDM and LPM values vary with test cut-off [10] and plotting these shows maxima similar to many of the other unitary tests considered in Chap. 4 (Fig. 5.1; Table 7.2).

Both LDM and LPM have a range of -1 (where Y or PSI $= -1$, Inacc $= 1$) to ∞ (Y or PSI $= + 1$, Inacc $= 0$). Since for diagnostic tests low values of NND and NNP and high values of NNM are desirable, higher values of LDM and LPM

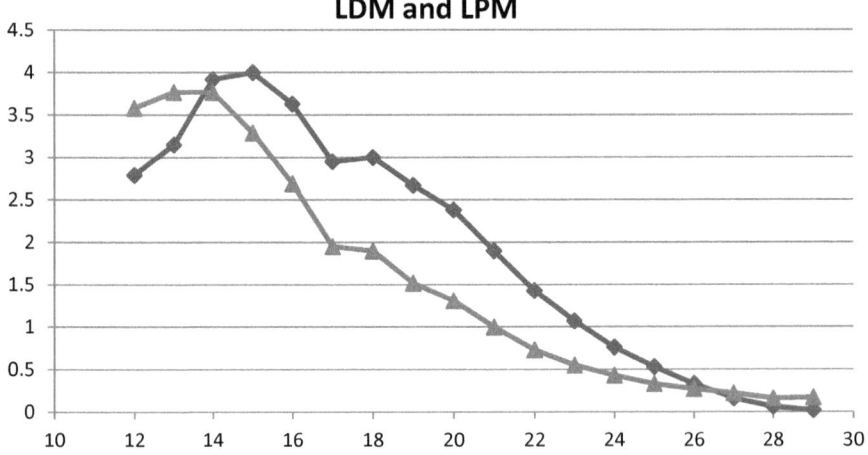

Fig. 5.1 Plot of likelihood to be diagnosed or misdiagnosed (LDM; diamonds) and likelihood to be predicted or misdiagnosed (LPM; triangles) on the y axis versus MACE cut-off (x axis) (adapted from [15])

(>1) would suggest a test more likely to favour correct diagnosis or prediction over misdiagnosis, whereas lower values of LDM and LPM (<1) suggest misdiagnosis is more likely than correct diagnosis or prediction. LDM values as high as ~7 have been recorded for tests which are both highly sensitive and specific ([14], p.75).

LDM and LPM should help clinicians and patients to evaluate potential risk–benefit trade-offs with particular diagnostic tests, and hence inform clinical decision making. For example, testing positive on a test with high LDM may permit a confident diagnosis, unlike the situation with a low LDM test, indeed the latter might be avoided for this very reason, especially if the test is expensive and/or poses risks to the patient.

The LDM formulations have found application in the evaluation of individual neurological signs and cognitive screening instruments [9, 10, 12–18, 33, 34] and also using data from meta-analyses of cognitive screening instruments [31, 33]. Nevertheless, LDM has shortcomings which are addressed in the development of the Efficiency Index (see Sect. 5.11).

5.8 Number Needed to Classify Correctly (NNCC)

Other "number needed" measures may be constructed from other test outcome measures. For example, the correct classification rate was defined as (Sect. 3.2.4):

$$\text{Correct classification rate} = \text{Sens} + \text{Spec}$$
$$= \text{TPR} + \text{TNR}$$
$$= Y + 1$$

Correct classification rate has a range 0–2, with higher values better.
From this, a "number needed to classify correctly" (NNCC) may be derived:

$$\text{NNCC} = 1/\text{classification rate}$$
$$= 1/(\text{Sens} + \text{Spec})$$
$$= 1/(Y + 1)$$

NNCC has a range from 0.5 to ∞, with lower values better.

Worked Example: Number Needed to Classify Correctly (NNCC)

In a screening test accuracy study of MACE [10], at the MACE cut-off of $\leq 20/30$, the sensitivity and specificity were 0.912 and 0.707 respectively (Sect. 2.2.1).

Hence the value for correct classification rate at this cut-off is (Sect. 3.2.4):

$$\text{Correct classification rate} = \text{Sens} + \text{Spec}$$

$$= 0.912 + 0.707$$
$$= 1.619$$

Hence the number needed for correct classification (NNCC) at this cut-off is:

$$NNCC = 1/(Sens + Spec)$$
$$= 1/(0.912 + 0.707)$$
$$= 0.618$$

From the MACE study data, $Y = 0.619$ (Sect. 4.2), and hence $NNCC = 1/(Y + 1) = 1/(0.619 + 1) = 0.618$ (NB it is entirely by chance that these values approximate the "golden ratio").

Referring to patients, NNCC is rounded up to the next whole integer and is therefore 1.

This measure is also pertinent to considerations of the ROC curve (Sects. 7.3.1 and 7.3.2).

5.9   Number Needed to Misclassify (NNMC)

The misclassification rate was defined (Sect. 3.2.4) as:

$$Misclassification\,rate = (1 - Sens) + (1 - Spec)$$
$$= FNR + FPR$$
$$= 1 - Y$$

Misclassification rate has a range 0–2, with lower values better.

From this, a "number needed to misclassify" (NNMC) may be derived:

$$NNMC = 1/Misclassification\,rate$$
$$= 1/(FNR + FPR)$$
$$= 1/(1 - Y)$$

NNMC has a range from 0.5 to ∞, with higher values better.

Worked Example: Number Needed To Misclassify (NNMC)

In a screening test accuracy study of MACE [10], at the MACE cut-off of $\leq$ 20/30, the FNR and FPR were 0.088 and 0.293 respectively (Sect. 2.2.2).

Hence the value for misclassification rate at this cut-off (Sect. 3.2.4) is:

$$\text{Misclassification rate} = \text{FNR} + \text{FPR}$$
$$= 0.088 + 0.293$$
$$= 0.381$$

Hence the number needed for misclassification (NNMC) at this cut-off is:

$$\text{NNMC} = 1/(\text{FNR} + \text{FPR})$$
$$= 1/(0.088 + 0.293)$$
$$= 2.62$$

From the MACE study data, $Y = 0.619$ (Sect. 4.2), and hence NNMC $= 1/(1 - Y) = 1/(1 - 0.619) = 2.62$.

Referring to patients, NNMC is rounded up to the next whole integer and is therefore 3.

This measure is also pertinent to considerations of the ROC curve (Sects. 7.3.1 and 7.3.2).

5.10 Likelihood to Classify Correctly or Misclassify (LCM)

Consideration of the numbers needed to classify correctly (NNCC; Sect. 5.8) and to misclassify (NNMC; Sect. 5.9) prompts development of a "likelihood to classify correctly or misclassify" (LCM) parameter, along the same lines as the characterisation of LDM and LPM (Sects. 5.6 and 5.7):

$$\text{LCM} = \text{NNMC}/\text{NNCC}$$
$$= (\text{Sens} + \text{Spec})/(\text{FNR} + \text{FPR})$$
$$= (\text{Sens} + \text{Spec})/(1 - \text{Sens}) + (1 - \text{Spec})$$

(Note the similarity of the last equation with one of the definitions of the diagnostic odds ratio, DOR (Sect. 2.4.1), substituting addition signs for multiplication signs.)

In terms of Y:

$$\text{LCM} = \text{NNMC}/\text{NNCC}$$
$$= (Y + 1)/(1 - Y)$$

Worked Example: Likelihood To Classify Correctly Or Misclassify (LCM)

In a screening test accuracy study of MACE [10], at the MACE cut-off of $\leq$ 20/30, the sensitivity and specificity were 0.912 and 0.707 respectively and the FNR and FPR were 0.088 and 0.293 respectively, giving values of NNCC and NNMC of 0.618 and 2.62 respectively.

Hence the value for LCM at this cut-off is:

$$LCM = NNMC/NNCC$$
$$= 2.62/0.618$$
$$= 4.24$$

From the MACE study data, $Y = 0.619$ (Sect. 4.2), and hence:

$$LCM = (Y + 1)/(1 - Y)$$
$$= (0.619 + 1)/(1 - 0.619)$$
$$= 1.619/0.381$$
$$= 4.24$$

Hence the test is more than 4 times more likely to classify correctly than to misclassify at this cut-off.

5.11   Efficiency Index (EI)

The "likelihood to be diagnosed or misdiagnosed" (LDM) measure (Sect. 5.6) has proved serviceable in evaluating a wide range of neurological signs and cognitive screening instruments used in the evaluation of disorders of cognition [9, 12–14, 31, 33]. Nevertheless, LDM has some limitations and shortcomings. Consistent with its ad hoc development, based on existing measures, LDM combined rates with different denominators (NNM, NND) which are not easily reconciled. Calculation of several parameters from the 2×2 contingency table is required to reach LDM (viz. Sens, Spec, Y, NND, Inacc, NNM), although ad hoc calculators exist [31]. Furthermore, the "number needed to diagnose" based on the Youden index (NND $= 1/Y$) incorporates considerations not only of diagnosis but also of misdiagnosis, since Sens $= (1 - FNR)$, and Spec $= (1 - FPR)$. The resulting LDM has boundary values of -1 (useless test: Sens $=$ Spec $= 0$, NND $= -1$; Inacc $= 1$, NNM $= 1$) and ∞ (perfect test: Sens $=$ Spec $= 1$, NND $= 1$; Inacc $= 0$, NNM $= \infty$), and so the LDM values cannot be easily accommodated, far less perfectly equated, with the qualitative classification scheme developed for likelihood ratios (Sect. 2.3.5) [6] which has boundary values of 0 and ∞ (Table 2.1), although LDM shares with LR an inflection point at 1 (LDM < 1 favours misdiagnosis, LDM > 1 favours diagnosis) [9, 13, 14].

A simple method to overcome these shortcomings of LDM has been proposed [19] by using NND* (Sect. 5.2) rather than NND as the denominator, whilst they share the same numerator (NNM). Just as LDM and LPM (Sects. 5.6 and 5.7) may be conceptualised as ratios of benefits (correct diagnosis, correct prediction) and harms (misdiagnosis), this new ratio might also justifiably be termed a "likelihood to be diagnosed or misdiagnosed"; however, to avoid confusion, an alternative name was deemed preferable. As Kraemer denoted (TP + TN) as "efficiency" ([7], p.27, 34, 115), so (FP + FN) might be termed "inefficiency" (see Sect. 1.3.1). Hence the ratio of efficiency/inefficiency may be denoted as the "efficiency index" (EI), thus [19]:

$$EI = NNM/NND^*$$
$$= (1/Inacc)/(1/Acc)$$
$$= Acc/Inacc$$

Alternatively, instead of EI, one might use the term "selectivity" since EI effectively selects true outcomes over false outcomes [22] (although this term might risk confusion with sensitivity and specificity).

In literal notation:

$$EI = (TP + TN)/(FP + FN)$$

In algebraic notation:

$$EI = (a + d)/(b + c)$$

Compare the simplicity of these literal and algebraic expressions of EI with the corresponding formulae for LDM (Sect. 5.6) and LPM (Sect. 5.7).

Like the Identification Index (II) (Sect. 4.6.1), EI takes into account both Acc and Inacc, but whereas Inacc is the divisor of Acc in EI, it is the subtrahend of Acc in II.

Since Acc and Inacc may be expressed in terms of Sens, Spec, P and P' so EI may also be expressed in terms of these measures:

$$EI = Sens \cdot P/Spec \cdot P'/(1 - Sens) \cdot P + (1 - Spec) \cdot P'$$

In error notation:

$$EI = (1 - \beta) \cdot P + (1 - \alpha) \cdot P'/(\beta \cdot P) + (\alpha \cdot P')$$

The boundary values of EI are 0 (useless test: Acc $= 0$; Inacc $= 1$) and ∞ (perfect test: Acc $= 1$, Inacc $= 0$), as for likelihood ratios.

Worked Examples: Efficiency Index (EI)

In a screening test accuracy study of MACE [10], at the MACE cut-off of $\leq$ 20/30, the absolute ("raw") values for NND* (Sect. 5.2) and NNM (Sect. 5.5) were 1.36 and 3.82 respectively.

Hence the value for EI at this cut-off is:

$$EI = NNM/NND^*$$
$$= 3.82/1.36$$
$$= 2.81$$

EI may also be calculated from the values of Acc and Inacc (Sect. 3.2.5), as:

$$EI = Acc/Inacc$$
$$= 0.738/0.262$$
$$= 2.81$$

EI may also be calculated from values of TP, FP, FN, and TN in the 2×2 contingency table (Fig. 2.2), as:

$$EI = (a + d)/(b + c)$$
$$= (104 + 453)/(188 + 10)$$
$$= 557/198$$
$$= 2.81$$

EI may also be calculated from values of Sens, Spec, P and P′:

$$EI = Sens \cdot P + \ Spec \cdot P'/(1 - Sens) \cdot P + (1 - Spec\ ) \cdot P'$$
$$= (0.912 \times 0.151)/(0.707 \times 0.849)/(0.088 \times 0.151) + (0.293 \times 0.849)$$
$$= 0.738/0.262$$
$$= 2.81$$

It is also possible to express EI in terms of the critical success index (CSI; see Sect. 4.8.1), or more precisely its complement, the Jaccard distance $(1 - CSI)$, since the denominator of that measure is given by "inefficiency":

$$1 - CSI = (FP + FN)/(TP + FN + FP)$$

$$= (FP + FN)/(N - TN)$$

Since EI = (TP + TN)/(FP + FN), then substituting gives:

$$EI = (TP + TN)/(1 - CSI) \cdot (N - TN)$$

Hence there is an inverse relation, such that the smaller the Jaccard distance, the larger EI.

In terms of CSI, this may be rearranged to read:

$$CSI = 1 - [(TP + TN)/(N - TN) \cdot EI]$$

Hence the larger EI, the smaller the subtrahend and hence the closer CSI is to unity. The factor relating and EI and CSI is given by:

$$EI.(1 - CSI) = (TP + TN)/(N - TN)$$

Worked Examples: Efficiency Index (EI) and Critical Success Index (CSI)

In a screening test accuracy study of MACE [10], where N = 755, at the MACE cut-off of $\leq 20/30$, TP = 104, TN = 453, and (1 − CSI) = 0.656 (Sect. 4.8.1).
Hence the value for EI at this cut-off is:

$$
\begin{aligned}
EI &= (TP + TN)/(1 - CSI).(N - TN) \\
&= (104 + 453)/(0.656).(755 - 453) \\
&= 557/0.656 \times 302 \\
&= 2.81
\end{aligned}
$$

CSI may also be calculated from these values:

$$
\begin{aligned}
CSI &= 1 - [(TP + TN)/(N - TN).EI] \\
&= 1 - [557/302 \times 2.81] \\
&= 1 - 0.656 \\
&= 0.344
\end{aligned}
$$

In terms of the 2×2 matrix, EI privileges neither criterion diagnosis nor test result, hence neither classifier (or explanatory variable) versus instance (or response variable). Hence, as such it may be conceptualised as a test of agreement, of criterion versus test result, and might also be construed as a measure of agreement, but different from the kappa statistic (Sect. 8.4.2) or Bland–Altman limits of agreement (Sect. 8.4.3).

Confidence intervals for EI may be calculated by applying the log method to data from the four cells of the 2 × 2 contingency table [21], as for likelihood ratios (Sect. 2.3.5) and diagnostic odds ratio (2.4.1).

Worked Example: Confidence Intervals for EI

In a screening test accuracy study of MACE [10], at the MACE cut-off of $\leq$ 20/30, as previously shown, EI = 2.81.

Hence the 95% confidence intervals (95% CI) for EI are [21]:

$$95\%\text{CI} = \left[1.96 \times \text{SE}\left(\log_e \text{EI}\right)\right]$$

$$\begin{aligned}\text{SE}\left(\log_e \text{EI}\right) &= \sqrt{[1/a - 1/(a+c) + 1/b - 1/(b+d)]} \\ &= \sqrt{[1/104 - 1/(114) + 1/188 - 1/(641)]} \\ &= 0.0678\end{aligned}$$

$$95\% \text{ CI} = 1.96 \times 0.0678 = 0.133$$

$$\text{EI} = 2.81 (95\% \text{ CI} = 2.46 - 3.21)$$

EI values may be classified qualitatively as for likelihood ratios [19], using the scheme of Jaeschke et al. [6] (Table 2.1), or as for diagnostic odds ratios, using the scheme of Rosenthal [29] (Sect. 2.4.1; demonstrated in [22]). EI values may be classified semi-quantitatively [19] using the heuristic of McGee [26], substituting EI for LR (Sect. 2.3.5; Table 2.1), such that approximately:

$$\text{Change in probability} = 0.19 \times \log_e(\text{EI})$$

EI values are dependent on P, and also vary with test cut-off (Fig. 5.2) [21]. A rescaled, quality EI (QEI) may also be calculated (Sect. 6.6.9).

EI has some advantages compared to other unitary measures [19]. Unlike Y (Sect. 4.2), MCC (Sect. 4.5), and II (Sect. 4.6.1), EI cannot have a negative value (boundary values 0, ∞). Both EI and DOR give optimistic results, DOR by choosing the best quality of a test and ignoring its weaknesses, particularly in populations with very high or very low risk. Ratios of DOR become unstable and inflated as the denominator approaches zero, which is also true of EI, although because the classes from the 2 × 2 contingency table are treated additively in EI rather than multiplicatively as in DOR the chance of denominator being zero is less.

Considering the cells of the 2 × 2 contingency table algebraically (Fig. 1.2), EI is less likely to be at boundary than DOR:

- If any one of a, b, c, or d = 0, then DOR will be at boundary (either 0 or ∞).

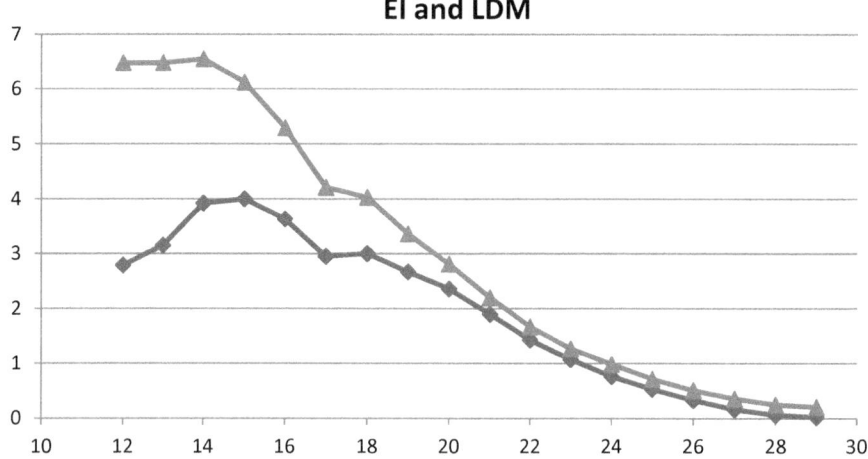

Fig. 5.2 Plot of efficiency index (EI; upper line, triangles) and of likelihood to be diagnosed or misdiagnosed (LDM; lower line, diamonds; as in Fig. 5.1) values (y axis) versus MACE cut-off score (x-axis) (adapted from [19])

- If any one of a, b, c, or d = 0, then EI will not be at boundary (either 0 or ∞).
- Even if two of a, b, c, or d = 0, then EI need not be at boundary (either 0 or ∞).
- Only if three of a, b, c, d = 0, then EI will necessarily be at boundary (either 0 or ∞).

EI shows the utility or inutility of diagnostic and screening tests, illustrating the inevitable trade-off between diagnosis and misdiagnosis. It may be a useful measure to communicate risk in a way that is easily intelligible for both clinicians and patients [19, 21, 22] and may be used to compare tests across different age-cohorts [23]. The EI measure may also be extended to balanced (Sect. 5.11.1), balanced level (Sect. 5.11.2), unbiased (Sect. 5.11.3) and quality (Sects. 6.6.9, 6.6.10 and 6.6.11) formulations.

5.11.1 Balanced Efficiency Index (BEI)

Balanced Accuracy (BAcc) has been defined (Sect. 3.2.6) as:

$$BAcc = (Sens + Spec)/2$$

Balanced Inaccuracy (BInacc) is its complement:

$$BInacc = 1 - BAcc$$
$$= (FNR + FPR)/2$$

Using BAcc and BInacc in place of Acc and Inacc, one may characterise a Balanced Efficiency index (BEI) [21] as:

$$\begin{aligned} \text{BEI} &= \text{BAcc}/\text{BInacc} \\ &= \text{BAcc}/(1 - \text{BAcc}) \\ &= (\text{Sens} + \text{Spec})/(1 - \text{Sens}) + (1 - \text{Spec}) \\ &= (\text{TPR} + \text{TNR})/(\text{FNR} + \text{FPR}) \end{aligned}$$

Hence unlike EI, BEI is independent of prevalence. Like EI, BEI has boundary values of 0 and ∞, with an inflection point at 1, where a value > 1 indicates correct classification and a value of < 1 indicates incorrect classification, such that values $\gg 1$ are desirable and a value of ∞ is an optimal classifier.

Worked Examples: Balanced Efficiency Index (BEI)

In a screening test accuracy study of MACE [10], at the MACE cut-off of $\leq$ 20/30, the sensitivity and specificity were 0.912 and 0.707 respectively and the FNR and FPR were 0.088 and 0.293 respectively.

Hence the value for BEI at this cut-off is:

$$\begin{aligned} \text{BEI} &= (\text{Sens} + \text{Spec})/(1 - \text{Sens}) + (1 - \text{Spec}) \\ &= (0.912 + 0.707)/(0.088 + 0.293) \\ &= 1.619/0.381 \\ &= 4.25 \end{aligned}$$

In this study, the values for BAcc and BInacc (Sect. 2.3.6) were 0.810 and 0.190 respectively.

$$\begin{aligned} \text{BEI} &= \text{BAcc}/\text{BInacc} \\ &= 0.810/0.190 \\ &= 4.25 \end{aligned}$$

Note how this differs from the value for EI (2.81) at this cut-off (Sect. 5.11).

5.11.2 Balanced Level Efficiency Index (BLEI)

Balanced Level Accuracy (BLAcc) has been defined (Sect. 3.3.3) as:

$$\text{BLAcc} = (\text{PPV} + \text{NPV})/2$$

Balanced Level Inaccuracy (BLInacc) is its complement:

$$BLInacc = 1 - BLAcc$$
$$= [(1 - PPV) + (1 - NPV)]/2$$
$$= (FDR + FRR)/2$$

It follows that Balanced Level Efficiency index (BEI) is given by [22]:

$$BLEI = BLAcc/BLInacc$$
$$= (PPV + NPV)/(1 - PPV) + (1 - NPV)$$
$$= (PPV + NPV)/(FDR + FRR)$$

Worked Examples: Balanced Level Efficiency Index (BLEI)

In a screening test accuracy study of MACE [10], at the MACE cut-off of $\leq$ 20/30, the PPV = 0.356 and NPV = 0.978 (Sect. 2.3.1); FDR = 0.644 and FRR = 0.022 (Sect. 2.3.2).

Hence the value for BLEI at this cut-off is:

$$BLEI = (PPV + NPV)/(FDR + FRR)$$
$$= (0.356 + 0.978)/(0.644 + 0.022)$$
$$= 1.334/0.666$$
$$= 2.00$$

In this study, the values for BLAcc and BLInacc (Sect. 3.3.3) were 0.667 and 0.333 respectively.

$$BLEI = BLAcc/BLInacc$$
$$= 0.667/0.333$$
$$= 2.00$$

Note how this differs from the value for EI (2.81) at this cut-off (Sect. 5.11).

5.11.3 Unbiased Efficiency Index (UEI)

Unbiased Accuracy (UAcc) has been defined (Sect. 3.2.7) as:

$$
\begin{aligned}
UAcc &= \left(Sens \cdot P + Spec \cdot P'\right) - \left(P \cdot Q + P' \cdot Q'\right)/1 - \left(P \cdot Q + P' \cdot Q'\right) \\
&= Acc - \left(P \cdot Q + P' \cdot Q'\right)/1 - \left(P \cdot Q + P' \cdot Q'\right)
\end{aligned}
$$

where P = prevalence and Q = the level or bias of the test.

Unbiased Inaccuracy (UInacc) is its complement:

$$
UInacc = 1 - UAcc
$$

Using UAcc and UInacc in place of Acc and Inacc, one may characterise an Unbiased Efficiency index (UEI) [21] as:

$$
\begin{aligned}
UEI &= UAcc/UInacc \\
&= UAcc/(1 - UAcc)
\end{aligned}
$$

Like EI, UEI has boundary values of 0 and ∞, with an inflection point at 1, where a value > 1 indicates correct classification and a value of < 1 indicates incorrect classification, such that values $\gg 1$ are desirable and a value of ∞ is an optimal classifier.

Worked Example: Unbiased Efficiency Index (UEI)

In a screening test accuracy study of MACE [10], at the MACE cut-off of $\leq 20/30$, the accuracy was 0.738 (Sect. 3.2.5), $P = 0.151$ and $Q = 0.387$ (Sect. 1.3.2), and hence UAcc = 0.378 and UInacc = 0.622 (Sect. 3.2.7).

Hence the value for UEI at this cut-off is:

$$
\begin{aligned}
UEI &= UAcc/UInacc \\
&= 0.378/0.622 \\
&= 0.608
\end{aligned}
$$

Note how this differs from the values for EI (2.81), BEI (4.25), and BLEI (2.00) at this cut-off (Sects. 5.11, 5.11.1, and 5.11.2).

The various formulations of EI (including QEI; see Sect. 6.6.9) are compared graphically in Fig. 5.3.

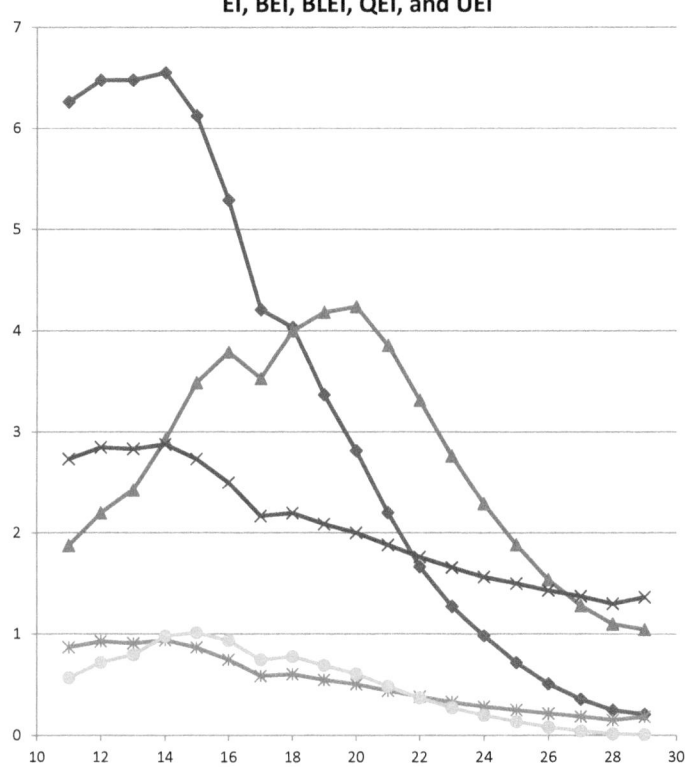

Fig. 5.3 Plot of EI (♦), BEI (▲), BLEI (×), QEI (*), and UEI (•) values (y axis) versus MACE cut-off score (x-axis) (adapted from [21] and [22]). For QEI, see Sect. 6.6.9

5.12 Number Needed for Screening Utility (NNSU)

The "number needed for screening utility" (NNSU) is the reciprocal or multiplicative inverse of SUI (Sect. 4.9) [12, 14]:

$$NNSU = 1/SUI$$
$$= 1/(PCUI + NCUI)$$
$$= 1/(Sens \times PPV) + (Spec \times NPV)$$

SUI ranges from 0 to 2 (Sect. 4.9). Hence NNSU ranges from ∞ (SUI = 0, no screening value) to 0.5 (SUI = 2, perfect screening utility), with low values of NNSU desirable. All NNSU values are positive (cf. NNS, Sect. 5.4). Following the qualitative classification of SUI (Sect. 4.9), it is also possible to classify NNSU values qualitatively. Generally, NNSU values may be dichotomised, as < 1 being acceptable or desirable, > 1 not so ("inadequate") [12, 14].

In literal notation:

$$NNSU = 1/TP^2[(TP + FN)(TP + FP)] + TN^2/[(TN + FP)(TN + FN)]]$$
$$= 1/[TP^2/p \cdot q] + [TN^2/p' \cdot q']$$

In algebraic notation:

$$NNSU = 1/[a/(a + c) \times a/(a + b) + d/(b + d) \times d/(c + d)]$$
$$= 1/a^2[(a + c).(a + b)] + d^2/[(b + d).(c + d)]$$

Worked Example: Number Needed For Screening Utility (NNSU)

In a screening test accuracy study of MACE [10], at the MACE cut-off of $\leq$ 20/30, PCUI = 0.325 and NCUI = 0.691 (Sect. 2.4.2).
   Hence the value for SUI (Sect. 4.9) is:

$$SUI = PCUI + NCUI$$
$$= 0.325 + 0.691$$
$$= 1.016$$

The value for NNSU is:

$$SUI = 1/SUI$$
$$= 1/1.016$$
$$= 0.984$$

This value of NNSU is qualitatively classified as adequate. As it refers to patients, NNSU is rounded up to the next whole integer and is therefore 1.

NNSU values vary with test cut-off [10]. A rescaled form may also be calculated (Sect. 6.6.12).

NNSU values have been calculated for many neurological signs and cognitive screening questions and instruments [10, 12, 14, 16–18].

5.13   Number Needed for Screening Disutility (NNSD)

A "number needed for screening disutility" (NNSD) may also be developed (first described in [20], p.109–10). NNSD is the reciprocal or multiplicative inverse of the summary disutility index (SDI) (Sect. 4.9):

$$NNSD = 1/SDI$$
$$= 1/(PCDI + NCDI)$$
$$= 1/[(FNR \times FDR) + (FPR \times FRR)]$$

SDI ranges from 0 to 2 (Sect. 4.9). Hence NNSD ranges from ∞ (SDI = 0, no screening disutility) to 0.5 (SDI = 2, maximum screening disutility), with high values of NNSD desirable. Generally, as for NNSU, NNSD values may be dichotomised, as > 1 being acceptable or desirable, < 1 not so.

Worked Example: Number Needed For Screening Disutility (NNSD)

In a screening test accuracy study of MACE [10], at the MACE cut-off of $\leq$ 20/30, PCDI = 0.057 and NCDI = 0.006 (Sect. 2.4.2).

Hence the value for SDI (Sect. 4.9) is:

$$SDI = PCDI + NCDI$$
$$= 0.057 + 0.006$$
$$= 0.063$$

The value for NNSD is:

$$NNSD = 1/SDI$$
$$= 1/0.063$$
$$= 15.87$$

This value of NNSD is qualitatively classified as adequate. As it refers to patients, NNSD is rounded up to the next whole integer and is therefore 16.

A rescaled form of NNSD may also be calculated (Sect. 6.6.13).

5.14 Likelihood for Screening Utility or Disutility (LSUD)

Consideration of the number needed for screening utility (NNSU; Sect. 5.12) and the number needed for screening disutility (NNSD; Sect. 5.13) prompts development of a "likelihood for screening utility or disutility" (LSUD) parameter:

$$LSUD = NNSD/NNSU$$
$$= [1/(PCDI + NCDI)]/[1/(PCUI + NCUI)]$$
$$= (1/SDI)/(1/SUI)$$
$$= SUI/SDI$$

Worked Example: Likelihood For Screening Utility Or Disutility (LSUD)

In a screening test accuracy study of MACE [10], at the MACE cut-off of $\leq$ 20/30, the number needed for screening utility (NNSU) was 0.984 (Sect. 5.12) and the number needed for screening disutility (NNSD) was 15.87 (Sect. 5.13).

Hence the value for LSUD at this cut-off is:

$$LSUD = NNSD/NNSU$$
$$= 15.87/0.987$$
$$= 16.13$$

$$LSUD = SUI/SDI$$
$$= 1.016/0.063$$
$$= 16.13$$

Hence the test is more than 16 times more likely to have screening utility than disutility at this cut-off.

5.15 Comparing Likelihood Measures

A number of likelihood measures have been considered in this chapter: LDM (Sect. 5.6), LPM (Sect. 5.7), LCM (Sect. 5.10), EI (Sect. 5.11), and LSUD (Sect. 5.14).

In the worked examples from the MACE study data, we find that LSUD (16.13) > LCM (4.24) > EI (2.81) > LDM (2.36) > LPM (1.28).

These measures will need to be examined at different cut-offs and in different datasets for firmer conclusions to be drawn, but the preliminary evidence suggests that LSUD is a very liberal measure, whilst LCM, EI, LDM, and LPM are more conservative measures.

References

1. Andrade C. Likelihood of being helped or harmed as a measure of clinical outcomes in psychopharmacology. J Clin Psychiatry. 2017;78:e73–5.
2. Citrome L, Ketter TA. When does a difference make a difference? Interpretation of number needed to treat, number needed to harm, and likelihood to be helped or harmed. Int J Clin Pract. 2013;67:407–11.
3. Cook RJ, Sackett DL. The number needed to treat: a clinically useful measure of treatment effect. BMJ. 1995;310:452–4.

4. Habibzadeh F, Yadollahie M. Number needed to misdiagnose: a measure of diagnostic test effectiveness. Epidemiology. 2013;24:170.
5. Hsieh S, McGrory S, Leslie F, Dawson K, Ahmed S, Butler CR, et al. The Mini-Addenbrooke's Cognitive Examination: a new assessment tool for dementia. Dement Geriatr Cogn Disord. 2015;39:1–11.
6. Jaeschke R, Guyatt G, Sackett DL. Users' guide to the medical literature. III. How to use an article about a diagnostic test. B. What are the results and will they help me in caring for my patients? JAMA. 1994;271:703–7.
7. Kraemer HC. Evaluating medical tests. Objective and quantitative guidelines. Newbery Park, California: Sage; 1992.
8. Larner AJ. Teleneurology by internet and telephone. A study of medical self-help. London: Springer; 2011.
9. Larner AJ. Number needed to diagnose, predict, or misdiagnose: useful metrics for non-canonical signs of cognitive status? Dement Geriatr Cogn Dis Extra. 2018;8:321–7.
10. Larner AJ. MACE for diagnosis of dementia and MCI: examining cut-offs and predictive values. Diagnostics (Basel). 2019;9:E51.
11. Larner AJ. Applying Kraemer's Q (positive sign rate): some implications for diagnostic test accuracy study results. Dement Geriatr Cogn Dis Extra. 2019;9:389–96.
12. Larner AJ. New unitary metrics for dementia test accuracy studies. Prog Neurol Psychiatry. 2019;23(3):21–5.
13. Larner AJ. Evaluating cognitive screening instruments with the "likelihood to be diagnosed or misdiagnosed" measure. Int J Clin Pract. 2019;73: e13265.
14. Larner AJ. Manual of screeners for dementia: pragmatic test accuracy studies. London: Springer; 2020.
15. Larner AJ. Defining "optimal" test cut-off using global test metrics: evidence from a cognitive screening instrument. Neurodegener Dis Manag. 2020;10:223–30.
16. Larner AJ. Mini-Addenbrooke's Cognitive Examination (MACE): a useful cognitive screening instrument in older people? Can Geriatr J. 2020;23:199–204.
17. Larner AJ. Mini-Cog versus Codex (cognitive disorders examination): is there a difference? Dement Neuropsychol. 2020;14:128–33.
18. Larner AJ. The "attended alone" and "attended with" signs in the assessment of cognitive impairment: a revalidation. Postgrad Med. 2020;132:595–600.
19. Larner AJ. Communicating risk: developing an "Efficiency Index" for dementia screening tests. Brain Sci. 2021;11:1473.
20. Larner AJ. The 2 × 2 matrix. Contingency, confusion and the metrics of binary classification. London: Springer; 2021.
21. Larner AJ. Evaluating binary classifiers: extending the Efficiency Index. Neurodegener Dis Manag. 2022;12:185–94.
22. Larner AJ. Efficiency index for binary classifiers: concept, extension, and application. Mathematics. 2023;11:2435.
23. Larner AJ. Cognitive screening in older people using Free-Cog and Mini-Addenbrooke's Cognitive Examination (MACE). Preprints.org. 2023;2023:2023040237. https://doi.org/10.20944/preprints202304.0237.v1
24. Laupacis A, Sackett DL, Roberts RS. An assessment of clinically useful measures of the consequences of treatment. N Engl J Med. 1988;318:1728–33.
25. Linn S, Grunau PD. New patient-oriented summary measure of net total gain in certainty for dichotomous diagnostic tests. Epidemiol Perspect Innov. 2006;3:11.
26. McGee S. Simplifying likelihood ratios. J Gen Intern Med. 2002;17:647–50.
27. Mitchell AJ. Index test. In: Kattan MW, editor. Encyclopedia of medical decision making. Los Angeles: Sage; 2009. p. 613–7.
28. Rembold CM. Number needed to screen: development of a statistic for disease screening. BMJ. 1998;317:307–12.
29. Rosenthal JA. Qualitative descriptors of strength of association and effect size. J Soc Serv Res. 1996;21:37–59.

30. Wald NJ, Morris JK. Two under-recognized limitations of number needed to treat. Int J Epidemiol. 2020;49:359–60.
31. Williamson JC, Larner AJ. "Likelihood to be diagnosed or misdiagnosed": application to meta-analytic data for cognitive screening instruments. Neurodegener Dis Manag. 2019;9:91–5.
32. Zermansky A. Number needed to harm should be measured for treatments. BMJ. 1998;317:1014.
33. Ziso B, Larner AJ. AD8: Likelihood to diagnose or misdiagnose. J Neurol Neurosurg Psychiatry. 2019;90:A20. https://jnnp.bmj.com/content/90/12/A20.1
34. Ziso B, Larner AJ. Codex (cognitive disorders examination) decision tree modified for the detection of dementia and MCI. Diagnostics (Basel). 2019;9:E58.

Chapter 6
Quality (Q) Measures

Contents

A. J. Larner, *The 2x2 Matrix*, https://doi.org/10.1007/978-3-031-47194-0_6

6.1   Introduction

In Chap. 1, the Q value developed by Kraemer [2] was discussed (see Sect. 1.3.2). Q is the probability of a positive test in the population examined, hence is known as the "positive sign rate" or the level of a test, or bias. Its complement, Q', is the "negative sign rate".

In literal notation (Fig. 2.1):

$$Q = (TP + FP)/N$$

In algebraic notation:

$$Q = (a + b)/N$$
$$= q/N$$

The probability of a negative test ("negative sign rate") in the population is the complement of Q, that is $1 - Q$ or Q'.

In literal notation:

$$Q' = (FN + TN)/N$$

In algebraic notation:

$$Q' = (c + d)/N$$
$$= q'/N$$

Taking into account the values of Q and Q' permits the calculation of "quality metrics". Kraemer specifically described "quality sensitivity" and "quality specificity", denoted QSN and QSP respectively [2].

Here a brief but comprehensive overview of these and other possible quality measures is given, expanding upon previous reports of quality measures [4, 7], along with worked examples (using the MACE dataset [5], as in previous chapters). The same classification of measures derived from Bossuyt is used as in previous chapters (viz. error-based, information-based, association-based) [1]. In the first edition of this book [7], subscript Q notation was used to denote quality measures, but this has now been eschewed in favour of an initial Q before each measure. Note that these Q measures should not be confused with the Q* index [3, 6] which is described elsewhere (Sect. 7.3.3).

In essence, all of these quality (or Q) measures give lesser values than their standard counterparts as a consequence of taking the values of Q and Q' into account. The use of these quality measures has not been widely adopted, but consideration should be given to using them to make evaluation of binary classifiers more rigorous, and less at risk of overoptimistic results.

6.2 Error-Based Quality Measures

6.2.1 Quality Sensitivity and Specificity (QSens, QSpec)

QSens and QSpec (equivalent to Kraemer's QSN and QSP [2], and denoted TPR_Q and TNR_Q, in the first edition of this book [7]) may be calculated to give the increment in each parameter beyond the level, such that:

$$QSens = (Sens - Q)/Q'$$

$$QSpec = (Spec - Q')/Q$$

QSens and QSpec range from 0 to 1, with higher values better, as for Sens and Spec.

Worked Example: QSens, QSpec

In a screening test accuracy study of MACE [5], at the cut-off of $\leq 20/30$ (Fig. 2. 2), Sens $= 0.912$ and Spec $= 0.707$ (see Sect. 2.2.1), and Q $= 0.387$ and Q' $= 0.613$ (Sect. 1.3.2).

Hence the value for QSens is:

$$\begin{aligned} QSens &= (Sens - Q)/Q' \\ &= (0.912 - 0.387)/0.613 \\ &= 0.857 \end{aligned}$$

The values for QSpec is:

$$QSpec = (Spec - Q')/Q$$
$$= (0.707 - 0.613)/0.387$$
$$= 0.242$$

Note how these quality measures differ from standard Sens (lower) and Spec (very much lower).

Like Sens and Spec, QSens and QSpec will vary with the chosen test cut-off. These calibrated, rescaled, or standardized indices of test parameters have been suggested to be more comparable across different samples [9]. Values of QSens and QSpec are generally inferior to the corresponding values of Sens and Spec [4].

6.2.2 Quality False Positive and False Negative Rates (QFPR, QFNR)

Quality false positive and false negative rates, QFPR and QFNR (previously FPR_Q and FNR_Q [7]), may be calculated based on their complementary relationship (Sects. 3.2.1 and 3.2.2) to QSpec and QSens respectively:

$$QFNR = 1 - QSens$$

$$QFPR = 1 - QSpec$$

Worked Examples: QFNR, QFPR

In a screening test accuracy study of MACE [5], at the cut-off $\leq 20/30$, QSens = 0.857 and QSpec = 0.242 (see Sect. 6.2.1).

Hence the values for QFNR and QFPR are:

$$QFNR = 1 - QSens$$
$$= 1 - 0.857$$
$$= 0.143$$

$$QFPR = 1 - QSpec$$
$$= 1 - 0.242$$
$$= 0.758$$

Note how these quality measures differ from standard FNR (0.088) and FPR (0.293) (Sect. 2.2.2).

6.2.3 Quality Accuracy, Inaccuracy (QAcc, QInacc)

One method to scale accuracy is to use the quality measures for Sens and Spec, QSens and QSpec (Sect. 6.2.1). The relationship of Acc to Sens and Spec is given by:

$$\text{Acc} = (\text{Sens.P}) + (\text{Spec.P}')$$

Substituting with values for QSens and QSpec, this becomes quality accuracy (QAcc):

$$\begin{aligned}
\text{QAcc} &= (\text{QSens.P}) + (\text{QSpec.P}') \\
&= [(\text{Sens} - Q)/Q'].P + [(\text{Spec} - Q')/Q].P'
\end{aligned}$$

Similarly, inaccuracy is given by:

$$\text{Inacc} = (\text{FNR.P}) + (\text{FPR.P}')$$

Substituting with values for QFNR and QFPR, this becomes quality inaccuracy (QInacc):

$$\begin{aligned}
\text{QInacc} &= (1 - \text{QSens}).P + (1 - \text{QSpec}).P' \\
&= (\text{QFNR.P}) + (\text{QFPR.P}') \\
&= 1 - \text{QAcc}
\end{aligned}$$

Worked Examples: Quality Accuracy and Inaccuracy (QAcc, QInacc)

In the screening test accuracy study of MACE [5], at the MACE cut-off of $\leq 20/30$, QSens = 0.857 and QSpec = 0.242 (Sect. 6.2.1) and QFNR = 0.143 and QFPR = 0.758 (Sect. 6.2.2).

Hence the value for quality Accuracy at this MACE cut-off is:

$$\begin{aligned}
\text{QAcc} &= (\text{QSens.P}) + (\text{QSpec.P}') \\
&= (0.857 \times 0.151) + (0.242 \times 0.849)
\end{aligned}$$

$$= 0.129 + 0205$$
$$= 0.335$$

Note how this differs from the calculations of Acc (= 0.738) and BAcc (0.810) at this cut-off, but approximates to UAcc (0.378) (see Sects. 3.2.5–3.2.7).

The value for quality Inaccuracy (QInacc) is:

$$QInacc = (QFNR.P) + (QFPR.P')$$
$$= (0.143 \times 0.151) = (0.758 \times 0.849)$$
$$= 0.022 + 0.644$$
$$= 0.665$$
$$= 1 - QAcc$$

Note how this differs from the calculations of Inacc (= 0.262) and BInacc (0.190) at this cut-off, but approximates to UInacc (0.622) (see Sects. 3.2.5–3.2.7).

Note that another method to scale accuracy (i.e. taking into account Q and Q') is the unbiased accuracy, UAcc (Sect. 3.2.7).

6.2.4   Quality Balanced Accuracy, Inaccuracy (QBAcc, QBInacc)

As shown in Sect. 6.2.3, quality accuracy (QAcc) is given by:

$$QAcc = (QSens.P) + (QSpec.P')$$

In the particular case where P = P' = 0.5, then, analogous to balanced accuracy (Sect. 3.2.6), this may be characterised as the quality balanced accuracy (QBAcc):

$$QBAcc = (QSens + QSpec)/2$$

Its complement is the quality balanced inaccuracy (QBInacc):

$$QBInacc = 1 - QBAcc$$
$$= (QFNR + QFPR)/2$$

Worked Examples: Quality Balanced Accuracy and Inaccuracy (QBAcc, QBInacc)

In the screening test accuracy study of MACE [5], at the MACE cut-off of $\leq$ 20/30, QSens $= 0.857$ and QSpec $= 0.242$ (Sect. 6.2.1).
    Hence the value for QBAcc at this MACE cut-off is:

$$QBAcc = (QSens + QSpec)/2$$
$$= (0.857 + 0.242)/2$$
$$= 0.5495$$

Just as BAcc (0.810) is greater than Acc (0.738) (see Sect. 3.2.6), so QBAcc is greater than QAcc (0.335).

$$QBInacc = 1 - QBAcc$$
$$= 1 - 0.5495$$
$$= 0.451$$

QInacc (0.665) is greater than QBInacc.

6.3   Information-Based Quality Measures

6.3.1   Quality Positive and Negative Predictive Values (QPPV, QNPV)

The rescaling of Sens and Spec according to the level of the test, Q, as QSens and QSpec (Sect. 6.2.1) may also be applied to other parameters, for example quality positive and negative predictive values, QPPV and QNPV (previously PPV_Q and NPV_Q [7]). Since, from Kraemer's [2] equations:

$$QSens = (Sens - Q)/Q' = (NPV - P')/P$$

and

$$QSpec = (Spec - Q')/Q = (PPV - P)/P'$$

rearranging it follows that:

$$QNPV = (QSens \times P) + P'$$

and

$$QPPV = (QSpec \times P') + P$$

This allows rescaled predictive values to be calculated at different levels of Q, as for Sens and Spec rescaled as QSens and QSpec [4].

Worked Examples: QPPV, QNPV

In a screening test accuracy study of MACE [5], at the cut-off $\leq$ 20/30, QSens = 0.857 and QSpec = 0.242 (see Sect. 6.2.1), and dementia prevalence in the patient cohort (N = 755) was P = 0.151 (Sect. 1.3.2).

Hence the values for QPPV and QNPV are:

$$
\begin{aligned}
QPPV &= (QSpec \times P') + P \\
&= (0.242 \times 0.849) + 0.151 \\
&= 0.356
\end{aligned}
$$

$$
\begin{aligned}
QNPV &= (QSens \times P) + P' \\
&= (0.857 \times 0.151) + 0.849 \\
&= 0.978
\end{aligned}
$$

These values are identical to the unscaled values of PPV and NPV (Sect. 2.3.1) because the same MACE cut-off was used, hence the positive sign rate Q = 0.387 (Sect. 1.3.2) was the same. If we select a different value of Q, say Q = Q' = 0.5, then:

$$
\begin{aligned}
QSens &= (Sens - Q)/Q' \\
&= (0.912 - 0.5)/0.5 \\
&= 0.824
\end{aligned}
$$

$$
\begin{aligned}
QSpec &= (Spec - Q')/Q \\
&= (0.707 - 0.5)/0.5 \\
&= 0.414
\end{aligned}
$$

Hence the values for QPPV and QNPV are now:

$$
\begin{aligned}
QPPV &= (QSpec \times P') + P \\
&= (0.414 \times 0.849) + 0.151 \\
&= 0.502
\end{aligned}
$$

$$QNPV = (QSens \times P) + P'$$
$$= (0.824 \times 0.151) + 0.849$$
$$= 0.973$$

With the change in Q and Q', QSens and particularly QNPV have changed little, reflecting the high sensitivity of MACE (few false negatives), whereas QSpec and QPPV have shown greater change (many false positives).

6.3.2 Quality False Discovery and False Reassurance Rates (QFDR, QFRR)

Quality false discovery and false reassurance rates, QFDR and QFRR, may be calculated based on their complementary relationship (Sect. 3.3.1 and 3.3.2) to QPPV and QNPV respectively:

$$QFDR = 1 - QPPV$$

$$QFRR = 1 - QNPV$$

Worked Examples: QFDR, QFRR

In a screening test accuracy study of MACE [5], at the cut-off $\leq 20/30$, QPPV $= 0.356$ and QNPV $= 0.978$ (see Sect. 6.3.1).
   Hence the values for QFDR and QFRR are:

$$QFDR = 1 - QPPV$$
$$= 1 - 0.356$$
$$= 0.644$$

$$QFRR = 1 - QNPV$$
$$= 1 - 0.978$$
$$= 0.022$$

These values are identical to the unscaled values of FDR and FRR (Sect. 2.3.2) because the same MACE cut-off was used, hence the positive sign rate $Q = 0.387$ (Sect. 1.3.2) was the same. If we select a different value of Q, say $Q = Q' = 0.5$, then QPPV $= 0.502$ and QNPV $= 0.973$ (Sect. 6.3.1).

Hence the values for QFDR and QFRR are now:

$$QFDR = 1 - QPPV$$
$$= 1 - 0.502$$
$$= 0.498$$

$$QFRR = 1 - QNPV$$
$$= 1 - 0.973$$
$$= 0.027$$

With the change in Q and Q', QFRR has changed very little whilst QFDR has shown greater change, commensurate with the effects on QNPV and QPPV (Sect. 6.3.1).

6.3.3   Quality Balanced Level Accuracy, Inaccuracy (QBLAcc, QBInacc)

Another method to scale accuracy (see Sect. 6.2.3 and 6.2.4) uses the balanced level accuracy (BLAcc; Sect. 3.3.3).

$$BLAcc = (PPV + NPV)/2$$

A quality balanced level accuracy (QBLAcc) may thus be calculated as:

$$QBLAcc = (QPPV + QNPV)/2$$

Its complement is the quality balanced level inaccuracy (QBLInacc):

$$QBLInacc = 1 - QBLAcc$$
$$= (QFDR + QFRR)/2$$

Worked Examples: Quality Balanced Level Accuracy and Inaccuracy (QBLAcc, QBLInacc)

In the screening test accuracy study of MACE [5], at the MACE cut-off of $\leq$ 20/30, QPPV = 0.356 and QNPV = 0.978 (Sect. 6.3.1).

Hence the value for QBLAcc at this MACE cut-off is:

$$QBLAcc = (QPPV + QNPV)/2$$
$$= (0.356 + 0.978)/2$$
$$= 0.667$$

$$QBLInacc = 1 - QBLAcc$$
$$= 1 - 0.667$$
$$= 0.333$$

Note that at this cut-off the values of QBLAcc and QBLInacc are equal to BLAcc and BLInacc (Sect. 3.3.3).

6.3.4 Quality Positive and Negative Likelihood Ratios (QPLR, QNLR)

Positive and negative likelihood ratios, being based on Sens and Spec, may be easily rescaled according to the level of the test, Q [4], as QPLR and QNLR (previously LR_Q+ and LR_Q- [7]) such that:

$$QPLR = QSens/(1 - QSpec)$$

$$QNLR = (1 - QSens)/QSpec$$

Worked Examples: QPLR, QNLR

In a screening test accuracy study of MACE [5], at the cut-off $\leq 20/30$, QSens $= 0.857$ and QSpec $= 0.242$ (see Sect. 6.2.1).
  Hence the values for QPLR and QNLR are:

$$QPLR = QSens/(1 - QSpec)$$
$$= 0.857/(1 - 0.242)$$
$$= 1.13$$

$$QNLR = (1 - QSens)/QSpec$$

$$= (1 - 0.857)/0.242$$
$$= 0.591$$

Note how these quality measures differ from standard PLR (3.11) and NLR (0.124) and hence the difference in their qualitative and quantitative classification (Sect. 2.3.5).

6.3.5   Quality Positive and Negative Predictive Ratios (QPPR, QNPR)

As for likelihood ratios (Sect. 6.3.4), so for positive and negative predictive ratios (Sect. 2.3.8):

$$QPPR = QPPV/(1 - QNPV)$$

$$QNPR = (1 - QPPV)/QNPV$$

Worked Examples: QPPR, QNPR

In a screening test accuracy study of MACE [5], at the cut-off $\leq 20/30$, QPPV $= 0.356$ and QNPV $= 0.978$ (see Sect. 6.3.1).

Hence the values for QPPR and QNPR are:

$$QPPR = QPPV/(1 - QNPV)$$
$$= 0.356/(1 - 0.978)$$
$$= 0.356/0.02159$$
$$= 16.49$$

$$QNPR = (1 - QPPV)/QNPV$$
$$= (1 - 0.356)/0.978$$
$$= 0.658$$

These values are identical to the unscaled values of PPR and NPR (Sect. 2.3.8) because the same MACE cut-off was used, hence the positive sign rate $Q = 0.387$ (Sect. 1.3.2) was the same. If we select a different value of Q, say $Q = Q' = 0.5$, then QPPV $= 0.502$ and QNPV $= 0.973$ (Sect. 6.3.1).

Hence the values for QPPR and QNPR are now:

$$QPPR = QPPV/(1 - QNPV)$$
$$= 0.502/(1 - 0.973)$$
$$= 18.59$$

$$QNPR = (1 - QPPV)/QNPV$$
$$= (1 - 0.502)/0.973$$
$$= 0.512$$

6.4 Association-Based Quality Measures

6.4.1 Quality Diagnostic Odds Ratio (QDOR)

As DOR is related to cut-off and hence Q, a rescaled DOR, QDOR (previously DOR_Q [7]), may also be calculated:

$$QDOR = QPLR/QNLR$$

Worked Example: QDOR

In a screening test accuracy study of MACE [5], at the cut-off $\leq20/30$, QPLR = 1.13 and QNLR = 0.591 (see Sect. 6.3.4).
Hence the value for QDOR is:

$$QDOR = QPLR/QNLR$$
$$= 1.13/0.591$$
$$= 1.912$$

Note how this quality measure differs from standard DOR (25.08) and hence the large change in its quantitative classification (Sect. 2.4.1).

6.4.2   Quality Positive and Negative Clinical Utility Indexes (QPCUI, QNCUI)

Rescaled clinical utility indexes (CUIs), QPCUI and QNCUI (previously CUI_Q+ and CUI_Q- [7]) may also be calculated. Initially this was formulated with only QSens and QSpec and standard PPV and NPV [4, 7] but logically both should be quality indices (this will amount to the same thing for a fixed cut-off). Hence:

$$QPCUI = QSens \times QPPV$$

$$QNCUI = QSpec \times QNPV$$

Worked Examples: QPCUI, QNCUI

In a screening test accuracy study of MACE [5], at the cut-off $\leq 20/30$, QSens $= 0.857$ and QSpec $= 0.242$ (Sect. 6.2.1) and QPPV $= 0.356$ and QNPV $= 0.978$ (Sect. 6.3.1).

Hence the values for QPCUI and QNCUI are:

$$\begin{aligned} QPCUI &= QSens \times QPPV \\ &= 0.857 \times 0.356 \\ &= 0.305 \end{aligned}$$

$$\begin{aligned} QNCUI &= QSpec \times QNPV \\ &= 0.242 \times 0.978 \\ &= 0.237 \end{aligned}$$

Note how these quality measures differ from standard PCUI (0.325) and NCUI (0.691) and hence the difference in their qualitative classification (Sect. 2.4.2).

6.4.3   Quality Positive and Negative Clinical Disutility Indexes (QPCDI, QNCDI)

Clinical disutility indexes (CDI), first described in the previous edition of this book ([7], p. 44–5), may also be rescaled as quality measures:

$$QPCDI = (1 - QSens) \times (1 - QPPV)$$
$$= QFNR \times QFDR$$

$$QNCDI = (1 - QSpec) \times (1 - QNPV)$$
$$= QFPR \times QFPR$$

Worked Examples: QPCDI, QNCDI

In a screening test accuracy study of MACE [5], at the cut-off $\leq$20/30, QFNR = 0.143 and QFPR = 0.758 (Sect. 6.2.2) and QFDR = 0.644 and QFRR = 0.022 (Sect. 6.3.2).

Hence the values for QPCDI and QNCDI are:

$$QPCDI = QFNR \times QFDR$$
$$= 0.143 \times 0.644$$
$$= 0.092$$

$$QNCDI = QFPR \times QFRR$$
$$= 0.758 \times 0.022$$
$$= 0.017$$

Note how these quality measures differ from standard PCDI (0.057) and NCDI (0.006). In this instance there are no changes in the suggested qualitative classification of these parameters (Sect. 2.4.3).

6.5   Unitary Quality Measures

Many of the measures considered in this section can be expressed in terms of Q (and P), as shown previously for Y (Sect. 4.2), PSI (Sect. 4.3), HMYPSI (Sect. 4.4), MCC (Sect. 4.5), critical success index (Sect. 4.8.1) and F measure (Sect. 4.8.3), so it might be argued that no further account of Q be taken. Nevertheless, the derived quality measures are worked through here.

6.5.1 Quality Youden Index (QY)

Quality Youden index, QY (previously Y_Q [7]), may be calculated based on its relationship to QSpec and QSens, such that [4]:

$$QY = QSens + QSpec - 1$$

Worked Example: Quality Youden Index (QY)

In a screening test accuracy study of MACE [5], at the cut-off $\leq 20/30$, QSens $= 0.857$ and QSpec $= 0.242$ (see Sect. 6.2.1).
  Hence the value for QY is:

$$QY = QSens + QSpec - 1$$
$$= 0.857 + 0.242 - 1$$
$$= 0.099$$

Note how this quality measure differs from standard Y (0.619) (Sect. 4.2).

6.5.2 Quality Predictive Summary Index (QPSI)

Quality predictive summary index, QPSI (or $Q\Psi$), may be calculated based on its relationship to QPPV and QNPV, such that [4]:

$$QPSI = QPPV + QNPV - 1$$

Worked Examples: Quality Predictive Summary Index (QPSI)

In a screening test accuracy study of MACE [5], at the cut-off $\leq 20/30$, QPPV $= 0.356$ and QNPV $= 0.978$ (see Sect. 6.3.1).
  Hence the value for QPSI is:

$$QPSI = QPPV + QNPV - 1$$
$$= 0.356 + 0.978 - 1$$
$$= 0.334$$

Note how this quality measure is identical to PSI (Sect. 4.3) because the same value of Q is being used.

If we select a different value of Q, say $Q = Q' = 0.5$, then QPPV $= 0.502$ and QNPV $= 0.973$ (Sect. 6.3.1).

Hence the value for QPSI is now:

$$QPSI = QPPV + QNPV - 1$$
$$= 0.502 + 0.973 - 1$$
$$= 0.475$$

6.5.3 Quality Harmonic Mean of Y and PSI (QHMYPSI)

The harmonic mean of Y and PSI (HMYPSI) was one of the new measures developed in the first edition of this book ([7], p. 78–81). A derived quality measure is given by:

$$QHMYPSI = 2/[1/QY + 1/QPSI]$$

Worked Example: Quality Harmonic Mean of Y and PSI (QHMYPSI)

In a screening test accuracy study of MACE [5], at the cut-off $\leq 20/30$, QY $= 0.099$ (Sect. 6.5.1) and QPSI $= 0.334$ (see Sect. 6.5.1).

Hence the value for QHMYPSI is:

$$QHMYPSI = 2/[1/QY + 1/QPSI]$$
$$= 2/[1/0.099 + 1/0.334]$$
$$= 0.153$$

Note how this quality measure differs from standard HMYPSI (0.433) (Sect. 4.4).

6.5.4   Quality Matthews' Correlation Coefficient (QMCC)

Matthews' correlation coefficient (MCC) is the geometric mean of Y and PSI. A derived quality measure is thus given by:

$$QMCC = \sqrt{(QY \times QPSI)}$$

Worked Example: Quality Matthews' Correlation Coefficient (QMCC)

In a screening test accuracy study of MACE [5], at the cut-off $\leq$20/30, QY = 0.099 (Sect. 6.5.1) and QPSI = 0.334 (see Sect. 6.5.2).

Hence the value for QMCC is:

$$
\begin{aligned}
QMCC &= \sqrt{(QY \times QPSI)} \\
&= \sqrt{(0.099 \times 0.344)} \\
&= 0.185
\end{aligned}
$$

Note how this quality measure differs from standard MCC (0.455) (Sect. 4. 5).

A quality normalised Matthews' correlation coefficient (QnMCC) might also be calculated:

$$
\begin{aligned}
QnMCC &= (QMMC + 1)/2 \\
&= (0.185 + 1)/2 \\
&= 0.593
\end{aligned}
$$

Note how this quality measure differs from standard nMCC (0.727) (Sect. 4. 5).

6.5.5   Quality Identification Index (QII)

Quality identification index, QII, may be calculated based on its relationship to QAcc and QInacc, such that:

$$
\begin{aligned}
QII &= QAcc - QInacc \\
&= QAcc - (1 - QAcc) \\
&= 2 \cdot QAcc - 1
\end{aligned}
$$

Worked Example: Quality Identification Index (QII)

In the screening test accuracy study of MACE [5], at the MACE cut-off of $\leq$20/30, QAcc = 0.335 and QInacc = 0.665 (Sect. 6.2.3).
  Hence the value for QII is:

$$QII = QAcc - QInacc$$
$$= 0.335 - 0.665$$
$$= -0.33$$

Note how this quality measure differs from standard II (0.475) (Sect. 4.6). As with II, a drawback of QII is that its value will be negative if QAcc is < 0.5.

6.5.6 Quality Critical Success Index (QCSI) and Quality F Measure (QF)

Rescaled quality formulations of these parameters (Sects. 4.8.1 and 4.8.3) may be easily calculated:

$$QCSI = 1/[(1/QPPV) + (1/QSens) - 1]$$
$$QF = 2/[1/QSens + 1/QPPV]$$

Worked Examples: QCSI, QF

In a screening test accuracy study of MACE [5], at the cut-off $\leq$20/30, QSens = 0.857 (Sect. 6.2.1) and QPPV = 0.356 (Sect. 6.3.1).
  Hence the values for QCSI and QF are:

$$QCSI = 1/[(1/QPPV) + (1/QSens) - 1]$$
$$= 1/[(1/0.356) + (1/0.857) - 1]$$
$$= 0.336$$

$$QF = 2/[1/QSens + 1/QPPV]$$
$$= 2/[1/0.857 + 1/0.356]$$
$$= 0.503$$

Since CSI is related to F by the equation F = 2CSI/(1 + CSI) (Sect. 4.8.3), then we would expect that:

$$QF = 2QCSI/(1 + QCSI)$$

If QCSI = 0.336, then substituting:

$$\begin{aligned} QF &= 2QCSI/(1 + QCSI) \\ &= 2 \times 0.336/(1 + 0.336) \\ &= 0.503 \end{aligned}$$

QED

Note how these quality measures differ from standard CSI (0.344) and F (0.512) (Sects. 4.8.1 and 4.8.3 respectively).

6.5.7   Quality Summary Utility Index and Summary Disutility Index (QSUI, QSDI)

Quality summary utility index, QSUI (previously SUI_Q [7]), may be calculated based on its relationship to QPCUI and QNCUI (Sect. 6.4.2) such that:

$$QSUI = QPCUI + QNCUI$$

Likewise, quality summary disutility index, QSDI, may be calculated based on its relationship to QPCDI and QNCDI (Sect. 6.4.3) such that:

$$QSDI = QPCDI + QNCDI$$

Worked Examples: QSUI, QSDI

In a screening test accuracy study of MACE [5], at the cut-off $\leq$ 20/30, QPCUI = 0.305 and QNCUI = 0.237 (Sect. 6.4.2) and QPCDI = 0.092 and QNCDI = 0.017 (Sect. 6.4.3).

Hence the values for QSUI and QSDI are:

$$\begin{aligned} QSUI &= QPCUI + QNCUI \\ &= 0.305 + 0.237 \\ &= 0.542 \end{aligned}$$

$$QSDI = QPCDI + QNCDI$$
$$= 0.092 + 0.017$$
$$= 0.109$$

Note how these quality measures differ from standard SUI (1.016) and SDI (0.063) and hence the changes in their qualitative classification (Sect. 4.9).

6.6 Quality Number Needed (Reciprocal) Measures and Their Combinations as Quality Likelihoods

6.6.1 Quality Number Needed to Diagnose (QNND and QNND*)

Quality number needed to diagnose (QNND and QNND*) may be calculated based on their relationship to QY and QAcc respectively:

$$QNND = 1/QY$$
$$QNND* = 1/QAcc$$

Worked Examples: QNND, QNND*

In a screening test accuracy study of MACE [5], at the cut-off $\leq 20/30$, QY $=$ 0.099 (Sect. 6.5.1) and QAcc $= 0.335$ (Sect. 6.2.3).
  Hence the values for QNND and QNND* are:

$$QNND = 1/QY$$
$$= 1/0.099$$
$$= 10.1$$

Referring to patients, NND is rounded up to the next whole integer and is therefore 11.

$$QNND^* = 1/QAcc$$
$$= 1/0.335$$
$$= 2.99$$

Referring to patients, NND* is rounded up to the next whole integer and is therefore 3.

Note how these quality measures differ from standard NND (1.62, rounded to 2) and NND* (1.36, rounded to 2) (Sect. 5.2).

6.6.2 Quality Number Needed to Predict (QNNP)

Quality number needed to predict (QNNP) may be calculated based on its relationship to QPSI:

$$QNNP = 1/QPSI$$

Worked Example: QNNP

In a screening test accuracy study of MACE [5], at the cut-off $\leq 20/30$, QPSI $= 0.334$ (Sect. 6.5.2).

Hence the value for QNNP is:

$$QNNP = 1/QPSI$$
$$= 1/0.334$$
$$= 2.99$$

Referring to patients, QNNP is rounded up to the next whole integer and is therefore 3. Note how this quality measure is identical to NNP (Sect. 5.3) because the same value of Q is being used.

If we select a different value of Q, say $Q = Q' = 0.5$, then QPSI $= 0.475$ (Sect. 6.5.2).

Hence the value for QNNP is now:

$$QNNP = 1/0.475$$
$$= 2.11$$

Referring to patients, QNNP is rounded up to the next whole integer and is therefore 3.

6.6.3 Quality Number Needed to Misdiagnose (QNNM)

Quality number needed to misdiagnose (QNNM) may be calculated based on its relationship to QInacc:

$$QNNM = 1/QInacc$$

Worked Example: QNNM

In a screening test accuracy study of MACE [5], at the cut-off $\leq$20/30, QInacc = 0.665 (Sect. 6.2.3).
   Hence the value for QNNM is:

$$QNNM = 1/QInacc$$
$$= 1/0.665$$
$$= 1.50$$

Referring to patients, QNNM is rounded up to the next whole integer and is therefore 2. Note how this quality measure differs from standard NNM (3.82, rounded to 4) (Sect. 5.5).

6.6.4 Quality Likelihood to Be Diagnosed or Misdiagnosed (QLDM)

Quality likelihood to be diagnosed or misdiagnosed (QLDM) (previously LDM_Q [7]) may be calculated based on its relationship to QInacc and QY, or to QNNM and QNND:

$$QLDM = (1/QInacc)/(1/QY)$$
$$= QNNM/QNND$$

Worked Example: QLDM

In a screening test accuracy study of MACE [5], at the cut-off $\leq$ 20/30, QInacc = 0.665 (Sect. 6.2.3) and QY = 0.099 (Sect. 6.5.1).
   Hence the value for QLDM is:

$$QLDM = (1/QInacc)/(1/QY)$$
$$= (1/0.665)/(1/0.099)$$
$$= 1.50/10.1$$
$$= QNNM/QNND$$
$$= 0.149$$

Note how this quality measure differs from standard LDM (2.36) (Sect. 5.6).

6.6.5 Quality Likelihood to Be Predicted or Misdiagnosed (QLPM)

Quality likelihood to be predicted or misdiagnosed (QLPM) may be calculated based on its relationship to QInacc and QPSI, or to QNNM and QNNP:

$$QLDM = (1/QInacc)/(1/QPSI)$$
$$= QNNM/QNNP$$

Worked Example: QLPM

In a screening test accuracy study of MACE [5], at the cut-off $\leq$20/30, QInacc = 0.665 (Sect. 6.2.3) and QPSI = 0.334 (Sect. 6.5.2).
  Hence the value for QLPM is:

$$QLPM = (1/QInacc)/(1/QPSI)$$
$$= (1/0.665)/(1/0.334)$$
$$= 1.50/2.99$$
$$= QNNM/QNNP$$
$$= 0.501$$

Note how this quality measure differs from standard LPM (1.27) (Sect. 5.7).

6.6.6 Quality Number Needed to Classify Correctly (QNNCC)

Quality number needed to classify correctly (QNNCC) may be calculated based on its relationship to QSens and QSpec, and hence QY:

$$QNNCC = 1/(QSens + QSpec)$$
$$= 1/(QY + 1)$$

Worked Example: QNNCC

In a screening test accuracy study of MACE [5], at the cut-off $\leq$ 20/30, QSens $= 0.857$ and QSpec $= 0.242$ (Sect. 6.2.1).

Hence the value for QNNCC is:

$$QNNCC = 1/(QSens + QSpec)$$
$$= 1/(0.857 + 0.242)$$
$$= 0.91$$

The value for QY $= 0.099$ (Sect. 6.5.1). Hence:

$$QNNCC = 1/(QY + 1)$$
$$= 1/(0.099 + 1)$$
$$= 0.91$$

Referring to patients, QNNCC is rounded up to the next whole integer and is therefore 1. Note how this quality measure differs from standard NNCC (0.618, rounded to 1) (Sect. 5.8).

6.6.7 Quality Number Needed to Misclassify (QNNMC)

Quality number needed to misclassify (QNNMC) may be calculated based on its relationship to QFNR and QFPR, and hence QY:

$$QNNCC = 1/(QFNR + QFPR)$$
$$= 1/(1 - QY)$$

Worked Example: QNNMC

In a screening test accuracy study of MACE [5], at the cut-off $\leq$20/30, QFNR $= 0.143$ and QFPR $= 0.758$ (Sect. 6.2.2).

Hence the value for QNNMC is:

$$QNNMC = 1/(QFNR + QFPR)$$
$$= 1/(0.143 + 0.758)$$
$$= 1.11$$

The value for QY $= 0.099$ (Sect. 6.5.1). Hence:

$$QNNMC = 1/(1 - QY)$$
$$= 1/(1 - 0.099)$$
$$= 1.11$$

Referring to patients, QNNMC is rounded up to the next whole integer and is therefore 2. Note how this quality measure differs from standard NNMC (2.62, rounded to 3) (Sect. 5.9).

6.6.8   *Quality Likelihood to Classify Correctly or Misclassify (QLCM)*

Quality likelihood to classify correctly or misclassify (QLCM) may be calculated based on its relationship to QNNCC and QNNMC, and hence QY:

$$QLCM = QNNMC/QNNCC$$
$$= [1/(1 - QY)]/[1/(QY + 1)]$$

Worked Example: QLCM

In a screening test accuracy study of MACE [5], at the cut-off $\leq$20/30, QNNCC $= 0.91$ and QNNMC $= 1.11$ (Sects. 6.6.6 and 6.6.7).

Hence the value for QLCM is:

$$QLCM = QNNMC/QNNCC$$
$$= 1.11/0.91$$

$$= 1.22$$

$$QLCM = [1/(1 - QY)]/[1/(QY + 1)]$$
$$= 1/(1 - 0.099)/1/(0.099 + 1)$$
$$= 1.22$$

Note how this quality measure differs from standard LCM (4.24) (Sect. 5.10).

6.6.9   Quality Efficiency Index (QEI)

Quality Efficiency Index (QEI) may be calculated based on the values of QAcc and QInacc [8]:

$$QEI = QAcc/QInacc$$

Worked Example: Quality Efficiency Index (QEI)

In the screening test accuracy study of MACE [5], at the MACE cut-off of $\leq 20/30$, QAcc $= 0.335$ and QInacc $= 0.665$ (Sect. 6.2.3).
   Hence the value for QEI is:

$$QEI = QAcc/QInacc$$
$$= 0.335/0.665$$
$$= 0.504$$

Note how this quality measure differs from standard EI (2.81) (Sect. 5.11), but is always positive, unlike QII (Sect. 6.5.5). This value of QEI approximates to, but is even more stringent than, that of unbiased EI (UEI $= 0.608$), and is less than the values of EI (2.81) or balanced EI (BEI $= 4.25$) (see Sects. 5.11–5.13). QEI is plotted against the range of MACE cut-offs in Fig. 5.3.

6.6.10   *Quality Balanced Efficiency Index (QBEI)*

Quality Balanced Efficiency index (QBEI) may be calculated based on the values of QBAcc and QBInacc:

$$QBEI = QBAcc/QBInacc$$

Worked Example: Quality Balanced Efficiency Index (QBEI)

In the screening test accuracy study of MACE [5], at the MACE cut-off of $\leq$20/30, QBAcc = 0.5495 and QBInacc = 0.451 (Sect. 6.2.4).
   Hence the value for QBEI is:

$$QBEI = QBAcc/QBInacc$$
$$= 0.5495/0.451$$
$$= 1.22$$

Note that QBEI is greater than QEI, just as BEI is greater than EI (see Sects. 5.11 and 5.11.1).

6.6.11   *Quality Balanced Level Efficiency Index (QBLEI)*

Quality Balanced Level Efficiency index (QBLEI) may be calculated based on the values of QBLAcc and QBLInacc:

$$QBLEI = QBLAcc/QBLInacc$$

Worked Example: Quality Balanced Level Efficiency Index (QBLEI)

In the screening test accuracy study of MACE [5], at the MACE cut-off of $\leq$ 20/30, QBLAcc = 0.667 and QBLInacc = 0.333 (Sect. 6.2.4).
   Hence the value for QBLEI is:

$$QBLEI = QBLAcc/QBLInacc$$
$$= 0.667/0.333$$
$$= 2.00$$

Note that QBLEI is equal to BLEI (Sect. 5.11.2) at this cut-off.

6.6.12   Quality Number Needed for Screening Utility (QNNSU)

Quality number needed for screening utility (QNNSU) (previously $NNSU_Q$ [7]) may be calculated based on the value of QSUI:

$$QNNSU = 1/QSUI$$

Worked Example: Quality Number Needed for Screening Utility (QNNSU)

In the screening test accuracy study of MACE [5], at the MACE cut-off of $\leq 20/30$, QSUI $= 0.542$ (Sect. 6.5.7).
   Hence the value for QNNSU is:

$$QNNSU = 1/QSUI$$
$$= 1/0.542$$
$$= 1.85$$

Referring to patients, QNNSU is rounded up to the next whole integer and is therefore 2. Note how this quality measure differs from standard NNSU (0.984, rounded to 1) (see Sect. 5.12).

6.6.13   Quality Number Needed for Screening Disutility (QNNSD)

Quality number needed for screening utility (QNNSD) may be calculated based on the value of QSDI:

$$QNNSD = 1/QSDI$$

Worked Example: Quality Number Needed for Screening Disutility (QNNSD)

In the screening test accuracy study of MACE [5], at the MACE cut-off of $\leq$ 20/30, QSDI = 0.109 (Sect. 6.5.7).
Hence the value for QNNSU is:

$$QNNSD = 1/QSDI$$
$$= 1/0.109$$
$$= 9.17$$

Referring to patients, QNNSD is rounded up to the next whole integer and is therefore 10. Note how this quality measure differs from standard NNSD (15.87, rounded to 16) (see Sect. 5.13).

6.6.14   Quality Likelihood for Screening Utility or Disutility (QLSUD)

Quality likelihood for screening utility or disutility (QLSUD) may be calculated based on the values of either QNNSU and QNNSD or QSUI and QSDI:

$$QLSUD = QNNSD/QNNSU$$
$$= QSUI/QSDI$$

Worked Example: Quality Likelihood for Screening Utility or Disutility (QLSUD)

In the screening test accuracy study of MACE [5], at the MACE cut-off of $\leq$ 20/30, QNNSU = 1.85 and QNNSD = 9.17 (Sects. 6.6.12 and 6.6.13).
Hence the value for QLSUD is:

$$QLSUD = QNNSD/QNNSU$$
$$= 9.17/1.85$$
$$= 4.96$$

Note that QLSUD is less than LSUD (16.13) (see Sect. 5.14).

References

1. Bossuyt PMM. Clinical validity: defining biomarker performance. Scand J Clin Lab Invest. 2010;70(Suppl242):46–52.
2. Kraemer HC. Evaluating medical tests. Objective and quantitative guidelines. Newbery Park, California: Sage; 1992.
3. Larner AJ. The Q* index: a useful global measure of dementia screening test accuracy? Dement Geriatr Cogn Dis Extra. 2015;5:265–70.
4. Larner AJ. Applying Kraemer's Q (positive sign rate): some implications for diagnostic test accuracy study results. Dement Geriatr Cogn Dis Extra. 2019;9:389–96.
5. Larner AJ. MACE for diagnosis of dementia and MCI: examining cut-offs and predictive values. Diagnostics (Basel). 2019;9:E51.
6. Larner AJ. Screening for dementia: Q* index as a global measure of test accuracy revisited. medRxiv. 2020. https://doi.org/10.1101/2020.04.01.20050567
7. Larner AJ. The 2 × 2 matrix. Contingency, confusion and the metrics of binary classification. London: Springer; 2021.
8. Larner AJ. Efficiency index for binary classifiers: concept, extension, and application. Mathematics. 2023;11:2435.
9. Larrabee GJ, Barry DTR. Diagnostic classification statistics and diagnostic validity of malingering assessment. In: Larrabee GJ, editor. Assessment of malingered neuropsychological deficits. Oxford: Oxford University Press; 2007. p. 14–26.

Chapter 7
Graphing Methods

Contents

7.1 Introduction

The methods of analysis of 2×2 contingency tables considered in the previous chapters of this book have all been arithmetical or algebraic (aside from brief mention of a graphical representation of sensitivity, specificity and predictive values; Sect. 2.3.4). Graphical depiction of test performance of binary classifiers is also possible. One of these performance graphing methods, the receiver operating characteristic (ROC) curve or plot, is widely used. It is also relevant to the definition of "optimal" test cut-offs which may in turn be used to calibrate test results when constructing 2×2 contingency tables (Sect. 1.5).

© The Author(s), under exclusive license to Springer Nature Switzerland AG 2024   187
A. J. Larner, *The 2x2 Matrix*, https://doi.org/10.1007/978-3-031-47194-0_7

7.2   Receiver Operating Characteristic (ROC) Plot or Curve

7.2.1   The ROC Curve or Plot

The receiver operating characteristic (ROC) curve or plot is a frequently used method to display the cumulated results of a quantitative test accuracy study [4, 11, 18, 24, 53, 55], which takes its origins from signal detection theory [37, 38].

In unit 2-dimensional ROC space, the Sensitivity (Sens), or "hit rate" or true positive rate (TPR), of the test is plotted on the ordinate (dependent variable) against false positive rate (FPR), the complement of Specificity (Spec), or (1 – Specificity), on the abscissa (independent variable) across the range of possible test scores with linear interpolation between points (an example is shown in Fig. 7.1 [26]). Empirically, this is a step function, tending to a curve as the number of instances, and hence points, approaches infinity. (Sometimes authors reverse the direction of the x-axis on the ROC plot, such that the origin coordinates become (1,0), and the abscissa thus plots specificity rather than false positive rate.)

The ROC plot is a graph of the relative trade-off of benefits, TPR (Sect. 2.2.1), against costs, FPR (Sect. 2.2.2), extending from conservative cut-offs (at bottom left, coordinates (0,0), Sens = 0, Spec = 1) to liberal cut-offs (at top right, coordinates (1,1), Sens = 1, Spec = 0). ROC plots ideally approximate the top left hand ("north west") corner of the ROC space (coordinates (0,1), Sens = 1, Spec = 1), corresponding to isosensitivity. In the situation where false positive rates are very low, it has been questioned whether ROC plotting is profitable ([51], p.153).

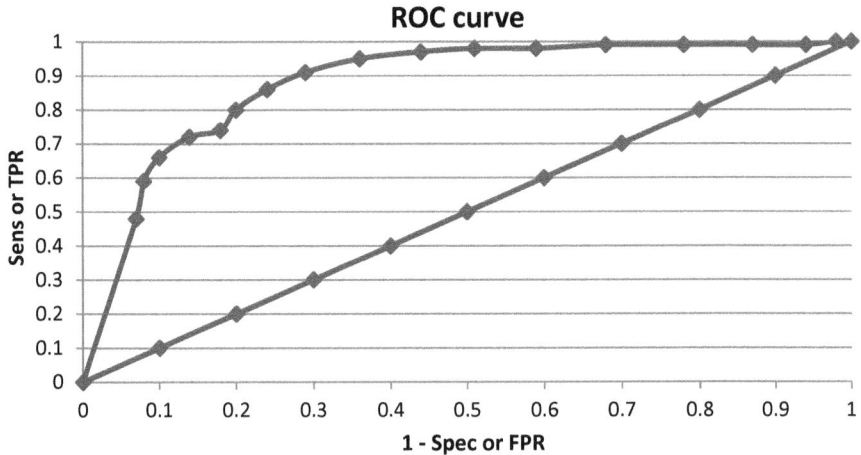

Fig. 7.1 Empirical ROC plot for diagnosis of dementia using the Mini-Addenbrooke's Cognitive Examination (MACE), with chance diagonal (y = x) (modified from [26]). TPR = true positive rate; FPR = false positive rate

ROC curves may be described as "threshold agnostic" or "threshold free" since test performance is shown without a specific threshold. ROC curves may also be used to define an optimal threshold (methods discussed below, Sect. 7.3). Moreover, as TPR and FPR are strict columnar ratios, algebraically independent of base rate, the ROC plot is insensitive to changes in class distribution.

ROC plots typically include the diagonal 45° line through ROC space ($y = x$, or Sens $= 1 -$ Spec, or TPR $=$ FPR) which represents the performance of a random classifier or the chance level (Fig. 7.1). This line also corresponds to a diagnostic odds ratio (DOR) $= 1$, indicative of a useless test, and reflective of the relationship between DOR and Sens and Spec (Sect. 2.4.1).

ROC curves which are symmetrical with respect to the anti-diagonal line through ROC space ($y = 1 - x$) have a constant DOR (isocontours, which might be termed "isoDORs"). Values of DOR range from 0 to ∞ (Sect. 2.4.1) and these limits are represented in the ROC plot: DOR $= \infty$ at the optimal ("north west") corner of the plot, running through coordinates (0,1) with $y = 1$ at the intersection with the ROC anti-diagonal; and DOR $= 0$ at the bottom right hand ("south east") corner of the plot, running through coordinates (1,0) with $y = 0$ at the intersection with the ROC anti-diagonal. Points below the diagonal 45° line through ROC space correspond to values of DOR <1 (this might be termed the "DOR 0-zone").

The slope of a tangent to the ROC curve at any point is equal to the likelihood ratio ($=$ TPR/FPR; Sect. 2.3.5) at that point [6], but the step function nature of most ROC plots makes it difficult to identify the point of maximum slope [13]. The slope is also related to the net harm to net benefit (H/B) ratio (Sects. 2.3.6 and 3.2.4), since:

$$\text{Net Harm (H)}/ \text{ Net Benefit (B)} = \text{Pre-test odds} \times \text{PLR}$$

where PLR $=$ positive likelihood ratio. Hence:

$$\text{Net Harm (H)}/ \text{ Net Benefit (B)} = (P/P') \times \text{PLR}$$
$$= (P/P') \times (\text{TPR/FPR})$$

and:

$$\text{Net Harm (H)/Net Benefit (B)} = C_{FP} - C_{TN}/C_{FN} - C_{TP}$$

Combining:

$$C_{FP} - C_{TN}/C_{FN} - C_{TP} = \text{Pre-test odds} \times \text{PLR}$$
$$= (P/P') \times \text{PLR}$$
$$= (P'/P') \times (\text{TPR}/\text{FPR})$$

and rearranging:

$$\text{PLR} = \text{TPR}/\text{FPR} = (C_{FP} - C_{TN}/C_{FN} - C_{TP}) \times (P'/P)$$
$$= H/B \times (P'/P)$$

7.2.2 Area Under the ROC Curve (AUC)

The area under the ROC curve (AUC) is the probability that a random person with disease has a value of the measurement above the cut-off compared to a random person without disease, or the percentage correct in a two-alternative forced choice task. This scalar value, also referred to as the concordance statistic or c-statistic, represents expected test performance and hence may be used as a measure of diagnostic accuracy (cf. other meanings of "accuracy", Sect. 3.2.5 [27, 33]).

The performance of a random classifier gives AUC $= 0.5$. If the confidence intervals of AUC (Sect. 1.7) overlap this value then the null hypothesis cannot be rejected. AUC < 0.5 is an outcome worse than random guessing. Various qualitative classification schemata for AUC values have been reported (Table 7.1) [4, 21, 41, 49, 52]. AUC values tend to be optimistic compared to other measures of "accuracy" [27].

Methods for calculation of AUC are mainly based on a non-parametric statistical test, the Wilcoxon rank-sum test, namely the proportion of all possible pairs of non-diseased and diseased test subjects for which the diseased result is higher than the non-diseased plus half the proportion of ties [10, 15, 16, 55, 56]. AUC may also be calculated from the DOR using the formula [50]:

$$\text{AUC} = \text{DOR}/(\text{DOR} - 1)^2 \cdot \left[(\text{DOR} - 1) - \log_e(\text{DOR})\right]$$

The latter may tend to overestimate AUC compared to the rank-sum method [28, 40].

Table 7.1 Some classifications of ROC plot AUC values

Metz [41] (1978):
- between 0.9–1.0: excellent
- 0.8–0.9: good
- 0.7–0.8: fair
- 0.6–0.7: poor
- 0.5–0.6: failed

Swets [49] (1988):
- ≥ 0.91: high accuracy
- 0.71–0.90: moderate accuracy
- 0.50–0.70: low accuracy

Jones and Athanasiou [21] (2005):
- ≥ 0.97: excellent
- 0.93–0.96: very good
- 0.75–0.92: good

Carter et al. [4] (2016):
- 0.90–0.99 excellent
- 0.80–0.89 good
- 0.70–0.79 fair
- 0.50–0.69 poor
- Reasonable ≥ 0.75

Yang and Berdine [55] (2017):
- >0.9: outstanding discrimination
- $0.8 \geq AUC > 0.7$: excellent discrimination
- $0.7 \geq AUC > 0.6$: acceptable discrimination
- $0.6 \geq AUC > 0.5$: poor discrimination
- 0.5: no discrimination

[*sic*, these "rule of thumb" rankings are discontinuous, as published]

Worked Example: AUC ROC Plot

The Mini-Addenbrooke's Cognitive Examination (MACE) [19], a brief cognitive screening instrument, was subjected to a screening test accuracy study in a large patient cohort, N = 755 [26]. From a ROC plot of the results (Fig. 7.1), AUC was calculated by rank-sum methods as AUC = 0.886, a value which may be qualitatively categorised as good [4, 21, 41] or moderate [49]. (NB this value uncategorised by Yang and Berdine schema [52], see Table 7.1.)

The MACE ROC plot is asymmetric (Fig. 7.1), so DOR varies with test cut-off, with a maximal value of 52.8 at MACE cut-off of $\leq 23/30$ [29]. AUC was calculated, at this maximal DOR [28], as [50]:

$$\begin{aligned} AUC &= DOR/(DOR-1)^2 \cdot \left[(DOR-1) - \log_e(DOR)\right] \\ &= 0.0197 \times 47.833 \\ &= 0.941 \end{aligned}$$

This is greater than the AUC value by rank-sum methods (0.886), presumably because the equation assumes a symmetric ROC curve with DOR = 52.8. The DOR-based AUC value may be qualitatively categorised as outstanding [52], excellent [4, 41], very good [21], or high accuracy [49]. Hence the categorisation of AUC has changed according to method of its calculation.

ROC plots, and specifically AUC, have some shortcomings in the measurement of test accuracy. The combination of test accuracy over a range of thresholds includes those which may be both clinically relevant and clinically nonsensical [39]. Hence only parts of ROC plots may be of clinical interest. Methods for partial ROC curve analysis are available [54]. A ROC plot may also be divided graphically to illustrate zones of test efficacy, the so-called zombie plot ("zones of mostly bad imaging efficacy" [46], although the technique is applicable to diagnostic tests other than imaging). It has been argued that AUC ROC should be replaced by the Matthews' correlation coefficient (MCC; Sect. 4.5) as the standard measure for assessing binary classification [5].

For a categorical classifier with n thresholds, there will be (n − 1) points in ROC space. Hence classifiers with a binary outcome produce a ROC dot rather than plot, and an area under a triangle rather than an area under a curve (Fig. 7.2).

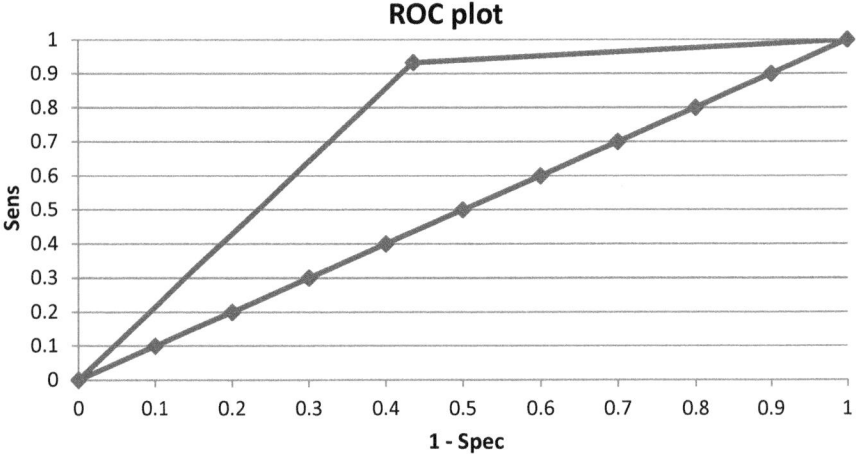

Fig. 7.2 ROC plot for a binary classifier: attended alone/attended with sign for the diagnosis of any cognitive impairment (dementia + MCI) versus no cognitive impairment, with chance diagonal (y = x) (data from [30], plot adapted from [40])

For the particular case of a binary classifier, it has been shown that the value of AUC also simplifies [43], to:

$$AUC = (Sens + Spec)/2$$

This, sometimes called "balanced accuracy" (Sect. 3.2.6), may also be expressed in terms of the Youden index, Y (Sect. 4.2):

$$Y = Sens + Spec - 1$$
$$Y + 1 = Sens + Spec$$

Substituting:

$$AUC = (Y + 1)/2$$

or:

$$Y = 2 \cdot AUC - 1$$

Whether ROC plots can be meaningfully applied in the assessment of binary categorical tests remains moot [40, 43].

Worked Example: AUC ROC Plot for Single Fixed Threshold

If MACE is treated as a binary classifier with a single fixed threshold of $\leq 20/30$ (based on maximal Youden index; Sect. 4.2), as shown in Fig. 7.3, AUC by rank-sum methods = 0.809. This may also be calculated from Sens = 0.912 and Spec = 0.707 at this MACE cut-off (Sect. 2.2.1):

$$\begin{aligned} AUC &= (Sens + Spec)/2 \\ &= (0.912 + 0.707)/2 \\ &= 0.809 \end{aligned}$$

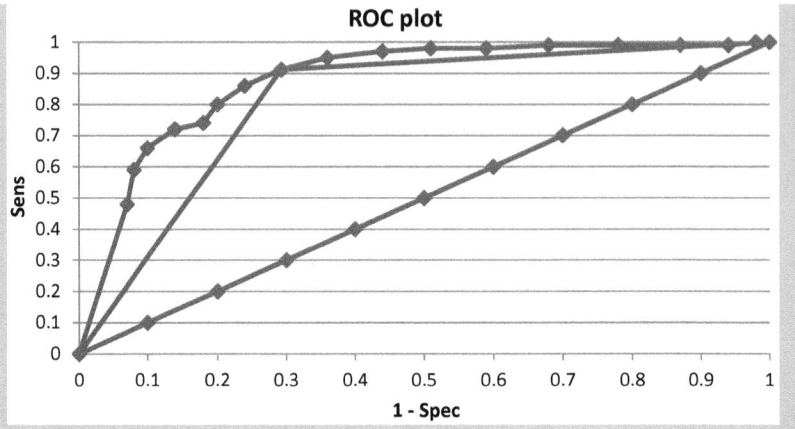

Fig. 7.3 ROC plot for MACE for the diagnosis of dementia versus no dementia, comparing MACE as a continuous scale (upper curve, = same as Fig. 7.1) or as a single fixed threshold binary classifier (lower triangle), with chance diagonal (y = x) (data from [26], plot adapted from [40])

AUC may also be calculated from the maximal Youden index at this threshold, which is 0.619 (Sect. 4.2):

$$AUC = (Y + 1)/2$$
$$= (0.619 + 1)/2$$
$$= 0.809$$

Hence, treating MACE as a binary classifier with a single fixed threshold underestimates AUC compared to the full ROC plot (= 0.886) [40].

AUC may also be calculated from DOR = 25.06 at this MACE cut-off:

$$AUC = DOR/(DOR - 1)^2 \cdot \left[(DOR - 1) - \log_e (DOR)\right]$$
$$= 0.0433 \times 20.839$$
$$= 0.902$$

This is greater than the AUC value calculated from Sens and Spec (0.809), presumably because the equation assumes the ROC curve to be symmetric with DOR = 25.06.

7.3   Defining Optimal Cut-Offs from the ROC Curve

One of the key functions of ROC plots is to permit the definition of "optimal" test cut-offs (Sect. 1.6). These various approaches are now considered. (Other methods for defining optimal cut-offs independent of the ROC plot are also available.)

7.3.1   Youden Index (Y)

As previously discussed (Sect. 4.2), Youden index (Y) is a global or unitary measure of test performance given by $Y = Sens + Spec - 1$.

The maximal value of Y corresponds to the point on the ROC curve which is the maximal vertical distance from the diagonal line ($y = x$) which represents the performance of a random classifier. Also known as c^*, this point minimizes misclassification (the sum of FPR and FNR) [1, 48]:

$$Y = max[Sens(c^*) + Spec(c^*) - 1]$$
$$= max Sens(c^*) - FPR(c^*)$$
$$= min[(FPR(c^*) + FNR(c^*))]$$

These equations also imply a minimization of the number needed to classify correctly (Sect. 5.8) and minimization of the number needed to misclassify (Sect. 5. 9).

In error notation:

$$Y = max[(1 - \beta) + (1 - \alpha) - 1]$$
$$= min[(\alpha + \beta)]$$

The cut-point maximising Sens and Spec is the point on the ROC curve which also represents the minimization of expected costs if and only if the cost of FN (misclassifying the diseased as undiseased) is equal to the cost of FP (misclassifying the undiseased as diseased) [22]. As previously discussed, this equivalence rarely if ever holds in clinical practice (Sect. 3.2.4).

In a study examining the Mini-Addenbrooke's Cognitive Examination (MACE) [19], optimal cut-off defined using the maximal Youden index was ≤ 20/30. This cut-off gave a relatively good balance of test sensitivity and specificity (Table 7.2) [26, 29].

Table 7.2 MACE sensitivity, specificity, and predictive values at optimal cut-off values as defined by various global parameters (data from [26, 28, 29, 31, 32, 34])

Optimal cut-off	Measure used to define optimal cut-off	Sens.	Spec.	Y	PPV	NPV	PSI
≤13/30	LPM (= NNM/NNP)	0.48	0.93	0.41	0.57	0.91	0.48
≤14/30	Acc LPM (= NNM/NNP) EI (= NNM/NND*)	0.59	0.92	0.51	0.56	0.93	0.49
≤15/30	CSI F measure HMYPSI MCC LDM (= NNM/NND) SUI Unbiased EI	0.66	0.90	0.56	0.53	0.94	0.47
≤18/30	Q* index (graphically)	0.80	0.80	0.60	0.42	0.96	0.38
≤ 19/30	Euclidean index (d)	0.86	0.76	0.62	0.38	0.97	0.35
≤20/30	Youden index (Y) Balanced EI	0.91	0.71	0.62	0.36	0.98	0.34
≤23/30	DOR Q* index (calculated)	0.98	0.49	0.47	0.25	0.99	0.24

Abbreviations: Acc = correct classification accuracy; CSI = critical success index; DOR = diagnostic odds ratio; EI = efficiency index; HMYPSI = harmonic mean of Y and PSI; LDM = likelihood to be diagnosed or misdiagnosed; MCC = Matthews' correlation coefficient; NND = number needed to diagnose; NNM = number needed to misdiagnose; NNP = number needed to predict; NPV = negative predictive value; PPV = positive predictive value; PSI = predictive summary index; Sens = sensitivity; Spec = Specificity; SUI = summary utility index; Y = Youden index

7.3.2   Euclidean Index (D)

The Euclidean index, d, is the point minimally distant from the top left hand ("north west") corner of the ROC plot, with coordinates (0,1), with the ROC intersect of a line joining these points designated c [7, 56], such that:

$$d = min\sqrt{\left[(1 - \text{Sens(c)})^2 + (1 - \text{Spec(c)})^2\right]}$$
$$= min\sqrt{\left[(\text{FNR(c)})^2 + (\text{FPR(c)})^2\right]}$$

Hence, Euclidean index is ideally zero; this will be seen to minimize the misclassification rate (Sect. 3.2.4). When c and c* (Sect. 7.3.1) do not agree, c* is deemed preferable since it maximizes the overall rate of correct classification ([54], p. 51–2).

In a study examining the MACE, optimal cut-off defined using the minimal Euclidean index was ≤ 19/30, giving a relatively good balance of sensitivity and specificity (Table 7.2) [29].

7.3.3 Q* Index

Using a summary ROC (SROC) curve based on data from meta-analyses, another index was proposed to determine optimal test cut-off: the Q* index. This is the point where the downward, negative, or anti-diagonal line through unit ROC space (y = 1 – x, or Sens = Spec, or Sens – Spec = 0, or TPR = 1 – FPR) intersects the ROC curve [42] (Fig. 7.4). Q* index may also be defined as the "point of indifference on the ROC curve", where the sensitivity and specificity are equal, or, in other words, where the probabilities of incorrect test results are equal for disease cases and non-cases (i.e. indifference between false positive and false negative diagnostic errors, with both assumed to be of equal value). For the particular case of a symmetrical ROC curve, Q* will be equal to the Euclidean index (d) [50].

Q* index has also been suggested as useful global measure of test accuracy [25], although its use for the comparison of diagnostic tests is controversial and has been generally discouraged [35].

As well as being assessed graphically, as the point of intersection of the ROC curve and the anti-diagonal through ROC space (Fig. 7.4), Q* index may also be calculated based on its relationship to the diagnostic odds ratio (DOR; Sect. 2.4.1). Q* may be calculated [50] as:

$$Q^* = \sqrt{DOR}/[1 + \sqrt{DOR}]$$

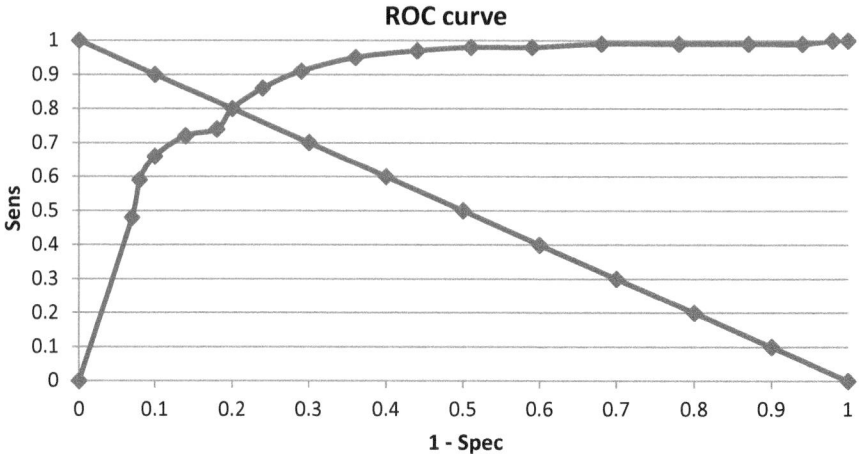

Fig. 7.4 ROC curve for diagnosis of dementia using MACE (= same as Fig. 7.1), intersecting with the anti-diagonal (y = 1 – x) line for assessment of Q* index (modified from [26])

Worked Example: Q* Index

A ROC plot of the results of the MACE study [26] intersected with the anti-diagonal line $(y = 1 - x)$ through unit ROC space, the Q* index, at 0.8 (Fig. 7.4), corresponding to an optimal MACE cut-off value of $\leq 18/30$, where Sens = Spec = 0.8.

Q* index was also calculated from DOR. The MACE ROC plot is not symmetric, so DOR varies with test cut-off, with a maximal value of 52.8 at MACE cut-off of $\leq 23/30$ [29].

Hence the value for Q* index [50] using this DOR was:

$$Q^* = \sqrt{DOR}/[1 + \sqrt{DOR}]$$
$$= \sqrt{52.8}/[1 + \sqrt{52.8}]$$
$$= 0.879$$

At this cut-off, Sens = 0.98 and Spec = 0.49, a poorer balance than seen with the graphical estimation of Q* index (Table 7.2) [28].

7.3.4 Other ROC-Based Methods

Other ROC-based methods to define optimal cut-off are described. In the "empirical method" [36], also known as the "product index" [14], a concordance probability maximizing the product of Sens and Spec is used. Another method uses the maximal "number needed to misdiagnose" [12] (Sect. 5.5) weighted according to an estimate of the relative costs of FN and FP test results [13].

7.3.5 Diagnostic Odds Ratio (DOR)

Maximal diagnostic odds ratio (DOR; Sect. 2.4.1) or its logarithm has frequently been used to define test cut-points. However, some authors have recommended against use of DOR because it produces a concave curve, and hence extremely high and low cut-points [3, 14]. Examining the MACE study data [29], maximal DOR cut-off ($\leq 23/30$) was an outlier compared to other ROC and non-ROC methods (as for Q* index calculated from DOR; Sect. 7.3.3 [28]), resulting in a high sensitivity but poor specificity test performance (Table 7.2).

7.3.6 Non-ROC-Based Methods

Various other global or unitary measures may be used to define test cut-off [29], for example maximal accuracy (Sect. 3.2.5) or kappa (Sect. 8.4.2), critical success index (Sect. 4.8.1) [32], F measure (Sect. 4.8.3), Matthews' correlation coefficient (Sect. 4.5), summary utility index (Sect. 4.9), the likelihood to be diagnosed or misdiagnosed (LDM; Sect. 5.6), the likelihood to be predicted or misdiagnosed (LPM; Sect. 5.7) [31], and the Efficiency Index (Sect. 5.11) [34].

In the study examining MACE, optimal cut-offs defined by these measures clustered around $\leq$ 13/30 to $\leq$ 15/30, resulting in greater specificity than sensitivity (Table 7.2) [29, 32].

7.4 Other Graphing Methods

A number of other graphing methods which display some of the measures derived from a 2 × 2 contingency table have been reported. None has achieved the breadth of usage of the ROC plot.

7.4.1 ROC Plot in Likelihood Ratio Coordinates

Johnson advocated transformation of ROC curves into positive and negative likelihood ratio (PLR, NLR; Sect. 2.3.5) coordinates, in part because half the potential region for ROC curves was deemed to have no meaning [20]. Test performance falling in the area below the diagonal is an outcome worse than random guessing; this has been termed the "perverse zone" [46] or the "DOR 0-zone" (Sect. 7.2.1).

Using logarithmic scales, optimal LR ROC curves bend further from the lower left corner, where $\log_{10}PLR = \log_{10}NLR = 0$, and towards the upper right ("north east") area where $\log_{10}PLR$ and $\log_{10}NLR$ approach infinity. The slope of the LR ROC curve equals the log diagnostic odds ratio at that point (whereas the slope of the ROC curve in its usual coordinates of Sens and 1 − Spec equals LR; Sect. 7.2.1). Using the transformed axes, AUC = 0 is a useless test, rather than 0.5 in the usual ROC plot. Comparison of tests is also possible using this method [20], as for regret graphs [17].

An attempt to convert data from the MACE study [26] to likelihood ratio coordinates is shown in Fig. 7.5 (compare with the conventional ROC plot of Fig. 7.1).

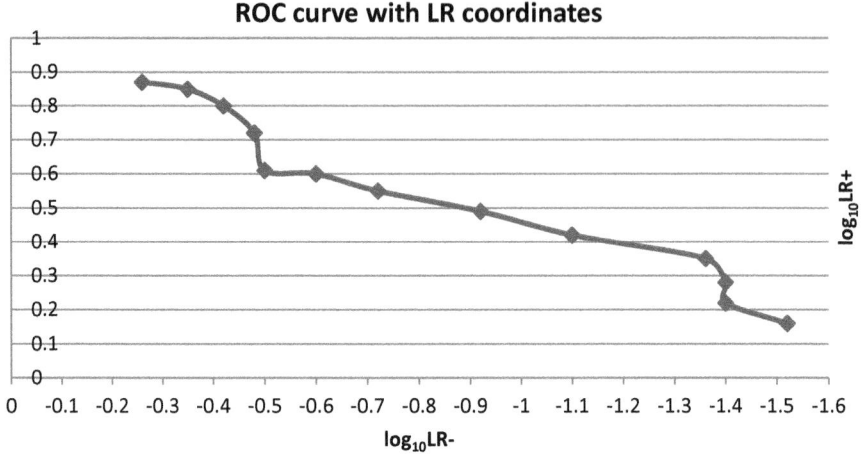

Fig. 7.5 ROC curve with LR coordinates for diagnosis of dementia using MACE (data from [26])

7.4.2 Precision-Recall (PR) Plot or Curve

The precision recall (PR) plot or curve is, like the ROC plot, a performance graphing method. It plots precision or positive predictive value (Sect. 2.3.1) on the ordinate against recall or sensitivity (Sect. 2.2.1) on the abscissa with linear interpolation between points [9] (Fig. 7.6).

This approach has both advantages and disadvantages. Like ROC curves, PR curves may be described as "threshold free" but they avoid some of the "optimism"

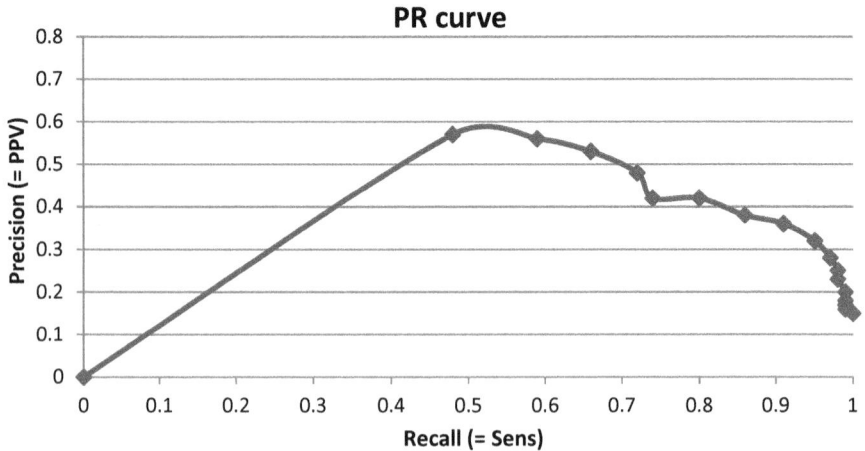

Fig. 7.6 Precision-recall (PR) plot or curve for diagnosis of dementia using MACE (modified from [26])

of ROC curves [8, 44] and are more informative than ROC curves when analysing skewed datasets [47]. On the down side, although area under the PR curve may be calculated this is not straightforward [23]. Visual interpretation may be adequate to denote better classification performance (as for ROC curves). The slope of a tangent to the PR curve at any point is equal to the ratio PPV/Sens, which does not correspond to any particular test measure (NB not to CSI [32]), unlike the situation with the ROC curve where the slope of a tangent at any point is equal to the likelihood ratio (= TPR/FPR). Overall, little use has been made of PR curves in assessing clinical diagnostic and screening tests [26].

7.4.3 Prevalence Value Accuracy Plots

Prevalence value accuracy contour plots attempt to include the cost of misclassifications (FP and FN; z-axis) as well as prevalence (x-axis) and unit cost ratio (y-axis) in graphing test performance. A derived misclassification index may give a different interpretation of the relative merit of tests compared to AUC ROC [45].

7.4.4 Agreement Charts

The agreement chart is a two-dimensional graph permitting visual assessment of the agreement or concordance between two observers. Unlike the kappa statistic (Sect. 8.4.2), the agreement chart helps to uncover patterns of disagreement between observers, but it can only be used for ordinal scale variables [2].

References

1. Baker SG, Kraemer BS. Peirce, Youden, and receiver operating characteristic curves. Am Stat. 2007;61:343–6.
2. Bangdiwala SI, Shankar V. The agreement chart. BMC Med Res Methodol. 2013;13:97.
3. Bohning D, Holling H, Patilea V. A limitation of the diagnostic-odds ratio in determining an optimal cut-off value for a continuous diagnostic test. Stat Methods Med Res. 2011;20:541–50.
4. Carter JV, Pan J, Rai SN, Galandiuk S. ROC-ing along: evaluation and interpretation of receiver operating characteristic curves. Surgery. 2016;159:1638–45.
5. Chicco D, Jurman G. The Matthews correlation coefficient (MCC) should replace the ROC AUC as the standard metric for assessing binary classification. BioData Mining. 2023;16:4.
6. Choi BC. Slopes of a receiver operating characteristic curve and likelihood ratios for a diagnostic test. Am J Epidemiol. 1998;148:1127–32.
7. Coffin M, Sukhatme S. Receiver operating characteristic studies and measurement errors. Biometrics. 1997;53:823–37.
8. Cook J, Ramadas V. When to consult precision-recall curves. Stata J. 2020;20:131–48.

9. Davis J, Goadrich M. The relationship between Precision-Recall and ROC curves. In: ICML '06: Proceedings of the 23rd International Conference on Machine Learning. New York:ACM; 2006. p. 233–40.

10. DeLong ER, DeLong DM, Clarke-Pearson DL. Comparing the areas under two or more correlated receiver operating characteristic curves: a nonparametric approach. Biometrics. 1988;44:837–45.

11. Fawcett T. An introduction to ROC analysis. Pattern Recognit Lett. 2006;27:861–74.

12. Habibzadeh F, Yadollahie M. Number needed to misdiagnose: a measure of diagnostic test effectiveness. Epidemiology. 2013;24:170.

13. Habibzadeh F, Habibzadeh P, Yadollahie M. On determining the most appropriate test cut-off value: the case of tests with continuous results. Biochem Med (Zagreb). 2016;26:297–307.

14. Hajian-Tilaki K. The choice of methods in determining the optimal cut-off value for quantitative diagnostic test evaluation. Stat Methods Med Res. 2018;27:2374–83.

15. Hanley JA, McNeil BJ. The meaning and use of the area under a receiver operating characteristic (ROC) curve. Radiology. 1982;143:29–36.

16. Hanley JA, McNeil BJ. A method of comparing the areas under receiver operating characteristic curves derived from the same cases. Radiology. 1983;148:839–43.

17. Hilden J, Glasziou P. Regret graphs, diagnostic uncertainty and Youden's index. Stat Med. 1996;15:969–86.

18. Hoo ZH, Candlish J, Teare D. What is an ROC curve? Emerg Med J. 2017;34:357–9.

19. Hsieh S, McGrory S, Leslie F, Dawson K, Ahmed S, Butler CR, et al. The Mini-Addenbrooke's Cognitive Examination: a new assessment tool for dementia. Dement Geriatr Cogn Disord. 2015;39:1–11.

20. Johnson NP. Advantages to transforming the receiver operating characteristic (ROC) curve into likelihood ratio co-ordinates. Stat Med. 2004;23:2257–66.

21. Jones CM, Athanasiou T. Summary receiver operating characteristic curve analysis techniques in the evaluation of diagnostic tests. Ann Thorac Surg. 2005;79:16–20.

22. Kaivanto K. Maximization of the sum of sensitivity and specificity as a diagnostic cutpoint criterion. J Clin Epidemiol. 2008;61:516–7.

23. Keilwagen J, Grosse I, Grau J. Area under precision-recall curves for weighted and unweighted data. PLoS ONE. 2014;9(3): e92209.

24. Krzanowski WJ, Hand DJ. ROC curves for continuous data. New York: CRC Press; 2009.

25. Larner AJ. The Q* index: a useful global measure of dementia screening test accuracy? Dement Geriatr Cogn Dis Extra. 2015;5:265–70.

26. Larner AJ. MACE for diagnosis of dementia and MCI: examining cut-offs and predictive values. Diagnostics (Basel). 2019;9:E51.

27. Larner AJ. What is test accuracy? Comparing unitary accuracy metrics for cognitive screening instruments. Neurodegener Dis Manag. 2019;9:277–81.

28. Larner AJ. Screening for dementia: Q* index as a global measure of test accuracy revisited. medRxiv. 2020. https://doi.org/10.1101/2020.04.01.20050567

29. Larner AJ. Defining "optimal" test cut-off using global test metrics: evidence from a cognitive screening instrument. Neurodegener Dis Manag. 2020;10:223–30.

30. Larner AJ. The "attended alone" and "attended with" signs in the assessment of cognitive impairment: a revalidation. Postgrad Med. 2020;132:595–600.

31. Larner AJ. Manual of screeners for dementia: pragmatic test accuracy studies. London: Springer; 2020.

32. Larner AJ. Assessing cognitive screening instruments with the critical success index. Prog Neurol Psychiatry. 2021;25(3):33–7.

33. Larner AJ. Accuracy of cognitive screening instruments reconsidered: overall, balanced, or unbiased accuracy? Neurodegener Dis Manag. 2022;12:67–76.

34. Larner AJ. Evaluating binary classifiers: extending the Efficiency Index. Neurodegener Dis Manag. 2022;12:185–94.

35. Lee J, Kim KW, Choi SH, Huh J, Park SH. Systematic review and meta-analysis of studies evaluating diagnostic test accuracy: a practical review for clinical researchers—Part II. Statistical methods of meta-analysis. Korean J Radiol. 2015;16:1188–96.

36. Liu X. Classification accuracy and cut point selection. Stat Med. 2012;31:2676–86.
37. Lusted L. Introduction to medical decision making. Springfield: Charles Thomas; 1968.
38. Lusted LB. Signal detectability and medical decision-making. Science. 1971;171:1217–9.
39. Mallett S, Halligan S, Thompson M, Collins GS, Altman DG. Interpreting diagnostic accuracy studies for patient care. BMJ. 2012;345: e3999.
40. Mbizvo G, Larner AJ. Receiver operating characteristic plot and area under the curve with binary classifiers: pragmatic analysis of cognitive screening instruments. Neurodegener Dis Manag. 2021;11:353–60.
41. Metz CE. Basic principles of ROC analysis. Semin Nucl Med. 1978;8:283–98.
42. Moses LE, Shapiro D, Littenberg B. Combining independent studies of a diagnostic test into a summary ROC curve: data-analytic approaches and some additional considerations. Stat Med. 1993;12:1293–316.
43. Muschelli J. ROC and AUC with a binary predictor: a potentially misleading metric. J Classif. 2020;37:696–708.
44. Ozenne B, Subtil F, Maucort-Boulch D. The precision-recall curve overcame the optimism of the receiver operating characteristic curve in rare diseases. J Clin Epidemiol. 2015;68:855–9.
45. Remaley AT, Sampson ML, DeLeo JM, Remaley NA, Farsi BD, Zweig MH. Prevalence-value-accuracy plots: a new method for comparing diagnostic tests based on misclassification costs. Clin Chem. 1999;45:934–41.
46. Richardson ML. The zombie plot: a simple graphic method for visualizing the efficacy of a diagnostic test. AJR Am J Roentgenol. 2016;207:W43-52.
47. Saito T, Rehmsmeier M. The precision-recall plot is more informative than the ROC plot when evaluating binary classifiers on imbalanced datasets. PLoS ONE. 2015;10(3): e0118432.
48. Schisterman EF, Perkins NJ, Liu A, Bondell H. Optimal cut-point and its corresponding Youden Index to discriminate individuals using pooled blood samples. Epidemiology. 2005;16:73–81.
49. Swets JA. Measuring the accuracy of diagnostic systems. Science. 1988;240:1285–93.
50. Walter SD. Properties of the summary receiver operating characteristic (SROC) curve for diagnostic test data. Stat Med. 2002;21:1237–56.
51. Weiskrantz L. Blindsight. A case study and implications (Oxford Psychology Series No. 12). Oxford: Clarendon Press; 1986.
52. Yang S, Berdine G. The receiver operating characteristic (ROC) curve. Southwest Respiratory Crit Care Chron. 2017;5(19):34–6.
53. Youngstrom EA. A primer on receiver operating characteristic analysis and diagnostic efficiency statistics for pediatric psychology: we are ready to ROC. J Pediatr Psychol. 2014;39:204–21.
54. Zhou XH, Obuchowski NA, McClish DK. Statistical methods in diagnostic medicine. 2nd ed. Hoboken, N.J: John Wiley; 2011.
55. Zou KH, O'Malley J, Mauri L. Receiver-operating characteristic analysis for evaluating diagnostic tests and predictive models. Circulation. 2007;115:654–7.
56. Zweig MH, Campbell G. Receiver-operating characteristic (ROC) plots: a fundamental evaluation tool in clinical medicine. Clin Chem. 1993;39:561–77.

Chapter 8
Other Measures, Other Tables

Contents

8.1 Introduction

The 2×2 contingency table may be used for purposes other than generating the various measures which have been discussed in Chaps. 2–7. These form a variegated assortment: combining results from more than one test; measures of association such as correlation coefficient, Cohen's d, and measures of agreement such as the kappa statistic; and other tables including higher order tables and other fourfold tables.

© The Author(s), under exclusive license to Springer Nature Switzerland AG 2024
A. J. Larner, *The 2x2 Matrix*, https://doi.org/10.1007/978-3-031-47194-0_8

8.2   Combining Test Results

If results are uncertain, further testing may be required for correct classification. When more than one test is undertaken, then methods to combine test scores may be required.

8.2.1   Bayesian Method

As previously mentioned in passing (Sect. 2.3.5), calculation of likelihood ratios provides a method for combining the results of multiple tests (1,2,...n), assuming the conditional independence of the tests in the presence and absence of the target diagnosis, by using Bayes' formula such that: Post-test odds

$$Post - test\ odds = Pre - test\ odds \times LR_1 \times LR_2 \times \ldots LR_n$$

Worked Example: Combining Tests, Bayesian method: MACE and SMC Likert Scale (1)

The Mini-Addenbrooke's Cognitive Examination (MACE) [24], a brief cognitive screening instrument, was subjected to a screening test accuracy study in a large patient cohort, N = 755 [37]. Some patients in this study (N = 129) were also administered a single-item cognitive screening question, the Subjective Memory Complaint (SMC) Likert Scale [49], in order to assess whether combining a patient-performance cognitive screener (MACE) with subjective memory evaluation (SMC Likert Scale) gave additional diagnostic information [36].

In the SMC Likert Scale, participants are asked: "In general, how would you rate your memory?" and given a choice of five possible responses: 1 = poor; 2 = fair; 3 = good; 4 = very good; 5 = excellent. SMC Likert Scale scores may be easily dichotomised: a score of 1 or 2 is categorised as SMC+, scores >2 as SMC− (i.e. higher scores better) [49].

Of the 129 patients administered both tests, MACE and SMC Likert Scale, 60 received a clinical diagnosis of cognitive impairment, hence pre-test probability (prevalence) of cognitive impairment in this cohort was 0.465, and pre-test odds were 0.869. Pre-test probability against disease was 69/129 = 0.535, and pre-test odds against disease were $(1 - 0.465)/0.465 = 1.15$ (see Sect. 1.3.3).

Using the MACE cut-off of ≤25/30 for cognitive impairment, established in the index study [24], PLR for a diagnosis of cognitive impairment was $p(R_i \mid D+)/p(R_i \mid D-) = (54/60)/(44/69) = 1.41$, a value producing only a slight increase in the probability of disease (Table 2.1). NLR for a diagnosis of no cognitive impairment was $(6/60)/(25/69) = 0.276$, a value producing a moderate increase in the probability of no disease (Table 2.1).

Using the SMC Likert Scale cut-off of ≤ 2, PLR for a diagnosis of cognitive impairment was $p(R_i \mid D+)/p(R_i \mid D-) = (42/60)/(60/69) = 0.805$, suggesting that subjective evaluation of memory actually slightly decreased the probability of a diagnosis of cognitive impairment (indeed it increases the probability of a diagnosis of functional cognitive disorder [7, 40]). NLR for a diagnosis of no cognitive impairment was $(18/60)/(9/69) = 2.3$, a value producing a moderate decrease in the probability of no disease (Table 2.1).

The results of the two tests, MACE and SMC Likert Scale, were combined using Bayes' formula:

$$\text{Post} - \text{test odds} = \text{Pre} - \text{test odds} \times \text{PLR}_{\text{MACE}} \times \text{PLR}_{\text{SMC}}$$
$$= 0.869 \times 1.41 \times 0.805$$
$$= 0.986$$

This can be converted back to a post-test-probability using the equation:

$$\text{Post} - \text{test probability} = \text{Post} - \text{test odds}/(1 + \text{post} - \text{test odds})$$
$$= 0.986/(1 + 0.986)$$
$$= 0.496$$

Thus, this combination of tests shows only a marginal improvement over the pre-test probability (0.465).

It is also possible to calculate the combined odds against disease using Bayes' formula:

$$\text{Post} - \text{test odds against} = \text{Pre} - \text{test odds against} \times \text{NLR}_{\text{MACE}} \times \text{NLR}_{\text{SMC}}$$
$$= 1.15 \times 0.276 \times 2.3$$
$$= 0.73$$

This can be converted back to a post-test-probability against disease using the equation:

$$\text{Post} - \text{test probability against} = 1/(1 + \text{post} - \text{test odds against})$$
$$= 1/(1 + 0.73)$$
$$= 0.578$$

Thus, this combination of tests shows a marginal increase over the pre-test probability against disease (0.535) (Larner, unpublished observations).

Worked Example: Combining Tests, Bayesian Method: AD8 and 6CIT (1) [44]

In the assessment of cognitive complaints, some authorities recommend the use of both a patient performance measurement and an informant interview before making a diagnosis of dementia. A previous study [32] in a dedicated cognitive disorders clinic examined both the informant AD8 scale [22] and the Six-item Cognitive Impairment Test (6CIT) patient performance cognitive screening instrument [10]. Both of these tests are negatively scored (i.e. higher scores = impairment worse).

Of the 177 patients administered both tests, 51 were diagnosed with dementia based on clinical diagnostic criteria, hence pre-test probability (prevalence) of dementia in this cohort was 0.288, and pre-test odds (Sect. 1.3.3) was 0.405.

Using the AD8 cut-off of $\geq 2/8$, PLR for a diagnosis of dementia was $p(R_i \mid D+)/p(R_i \mid D-) = (49/51)/(112/126) = 1.08$, a value producing only a slight increase in the probability of dementia (Table 2.1), notwithstanding its very high sensitivity.

Using the 6CIT cut-off of $\geq 8/28$, PLR for a diagnosis of dementia was $p(R_i \mid D+)/p(R_i \mid D-) = (44/51)/(48/126) = 2.26$, a value producing a moderate increase in the probability of dementia (Table 2.1).

The results of the two tests were combined using Bayes' formula:

$$\text{Post} - \text{test odds} = \text{Pre} - \text{test odds} \times \text{PLR}_{AD8} \times \text{PLR}_{6CIT}$$
$$= 0.405 \times 1.08 \times 2.26$$
$$= 0.988$$

This can be converted back to a post-test-probability using the equation:

$$\text{Post} - \text{test probability} = \text{Post} - \text{test odds}/(1 + \text{post} - \text{test odds})$$
$$= 0.988/(1 + 0.988)$$
$$= 0.497$$

This combination of tests therefore shows improvement compared to the pre-test probability of 0.288.

8.2.2 Boolean Method: "AND" and "OR" Logical Operators

The Bayesian method for combining test results may be compared with combination using a Boolean method based on simple logical rules, connectives, or operators ([38], p. 81–2, 133–6).

The mathematician George Boole (1815–64) defined three simple logical rules: the AND, OR, and NOT operators. The latter has previously been encountered in the characterization of paired complementary measures (Sect. 3.1). Using the "AND" and "OR" rules, one may construct tables akin to the truth tables developed for use in logic by Wittgenstein for the "and" and "or" connectives used to determine the truth or falsity of simple propositions (Fig. 8.1), perhaps one of Wittgenstein's most valuable if unwitting contributions to neurology and neuroscience [45].

Considering the 2×2 matrix, combination of two test results using the "AND" rule requires both tests to be positive for the target diagnosis to be made, i.e. any combination other than both tests positive is considered to rule out the diagnosis, an approach which privileges identification of true and false positives (Fig. 8.2a). This is sometimes known as series, serial or conjunctive combination, "believe the negative", or sequency (the first of these terms is avoided here as ambiguous, sometimes being used to refer to the situation where performance of a second test is dependent on the outcome of the first test, rather than all tests being performed on all subjects regardless of the result of the first).

Combination of two test results using the "OR" rule permits diagnosis to be made if either test is positive, i.e. any combination other than both tests negative is considered to rule in the diagnosis, an approach which privileges identification of true and false negatives (Fig. 8.2b). This is sometimes known as parallel or compensatory combination, "believe the positive", or simultaneity.

Evidently the "AND" criterion is more severe, and preferable if false positive (FP) outcomes are particularly to be avoided, whilst the "OR" criterion is more liberal and preferable if false negative (FN) outcomes are particularly undesirable.

a) "and"

Classifier diagnosis			
Test 1	Test 2	Test 3	Test 1 "and" Test 2
D+	D+	-	D+
D+	D-	-	D-
D-	D+	-	D-
D-	D-	-	D-
			Test 1 "and" Test 2 "and" Test 3
D+	D+	D+	D+
D+	D+	D-	D-
D+	D-	D+	D-
D-	D+	D+	D-
D+	D-	D-	D-
D-	D+	D-	D-
D-	D-	D+	D-
D-	D-	D-	D-

b) "or"

Classifier diagnosis			
Test 1	Test 2	Test 3	Test 1 "or" Test 2
D+	D+	-	D+
D+	D-	-	D+
D-	D+	-	D+
D-	D-	-	D-
			Test 1 "or" Test 2 "or" Test 3
D+	D+	D+	D+
D+	D+	D-	D+
D+	D-	D+	D+
D-	D+	D+	D+
D+	D-	D-	D+
D-	D+	D-	D+
D-	D-	D+	D+
D-	D-	D-	D-

Fig. 8.1 Truth tables for simple logical rules of combination for 2 or 3 tests: a) "and"; b) "or"

a) "and"

		Test 1	
		Positive	**Negative**
Test 2	**Positive**	+	-
	Negative	-	-

b) "or"

		Test 1	
		Positive	**Negative**
Test 2	**Positive**	+	+
	Negative	+	-

Fig. 8.2 2 × 2 contingency tables incorporating Boolean operators: a) "and"; b) "or". The former corresponds to a binary multiplication table

Worked Example: Combining Tests, Boolean Method: MACE and SMC Likert Scale (2)

MACE and SMC Likert results [36] were combined in series: both tests were required to be positive (MACE ≤25/30 and SMC ≤2) for the target diagnosis of cognitive impairment to be made. This permitted the construction of a 2 × 2 contingency table accommodating both tests (Fig. 8.3a).

a)

		Diagnosis	
		Cognitive impairment present	**Cognitive impairment absent**
MACE "AND" SMC outcome	**≤25/30 and ≤2**	True positive [TP] = **40**	False positive [FP] = **40**
	≤25/30 and >2, or >25/30	False negative [FN] = **20**	True negative [TN] = **29**

b)

		Diagnosis	
		Cognitive impairment present	**Cognitive impairment absent**
MACE "OR" SMC outcome	**≤25/30 or ≤2**	True positive [TP] = **56**	False positive [FP] = **64**
	>25/30 and >2	False negative [FN] = **4**	True negative [TN] = **5**

Fig. 8.3 2 × 2 contingency tables for combination of Mini-Addenbrooke's Cognitive Examination (MACE) and SMC Likert Scale outcomes (N = 129) for the diagnosis of cognitive impairment: a) "AND" rule, series combination; b) "OR" rule, parallel combination (data from [36])

From the combined 2 × 2 contingency table, the positive predictive value may be calculated as TP/(TP + FP) = 40/ (40 + 40) = 0.5, similar to the post-test-probability value obtained using the Bayesian method (Sect. 8.2.1) based on multiplication of pre-test odds and individual test LRs (0.496).

The negative predictive value may be calculated as TN/(FN + TN) = 29/ (20 + 29) = 0.59, similar to the post-test-probability against (0.578) (Larner, unpublished observations).

Worked Example: Combining Tests, Boolean Method: AD8 and 6CIT (2) [44]

The Boolean method was applied to the data from the study examining both the informant AD8 scale and the Six-item Cognitive Impairment Test (6CIT) patient performance cognitive screening instrument [32].

Combination using the simple logical "AND" rule (series combination or sequence) required both tests to be positive (AD8 ≥2/8 and 6CIT ≥8/28) for the target diagnosis of dementia to be made. This permitted the construction of a 2 × 2 contingency table accommodating both tests (Fig. 8.4).

		Diagnosis	
		Dementia present	**Dementia absent**
AD8 "AND"	≥2/8 and ≥8/28	True positive [TP] = 42	False positive [FP] = 45
6CIT outcome	≥2/8 and >8/28, or <2/8	False negative [FN] = 9	True negative [TN] = 81

Fig. 8.4 2 × 2 contingency table for series combination of informant Ascertain Dementia 8 (AD8) "AND" Six-item Cognitive Impairment Test (6CIT) outcomes (N = 177) for the diagnosis of dementia (data updated from [32])

From the contingency table, the positive predictive value may be calculated as TP/(TP + FP) = 42/ (42 + 45) = 0.483, similar to the post-test-probability (0.497) value obtained using the Bayesian method based on multiplication of pre-test odds and individual test LRs (Sect. 8.2.1) (Larner, unpublished observations).

It is also possible to calculate Sens and Spec for two tests (Test 1, Test 2) applied in series ("AND") or in parallel ("OR") based on individual test Sens and Spec using the equations:

$$\text{Sens}_{1\text{"AND"}2} = \text{Sens}_1 \times \text{Sens}_2$$

$$\text{Spec}_{1\text{"AND"}2} = \text{Spec}_1 + \left[\left(1 - \text{Spec}_1\right) \times \text{Spec}_2\right]$$
$$= \text{Spec}_1 + \text{Spec}_2 - \left[\text{Spec}_1 \times \text{Spec}_2\right]$$

$$\text{Sens}_{1\text{"OR"}2} = \text{Sens}_1 + [(1 - \text{Sens}_1) \times \text{Sens}_2]$$
$$= \text{Sens}_1 + \text{Sens}_2 - [\text{Sens}_1 \times \text{Sens}_2]$$

$$\text{Spec}_{1\text{"OR"}2} = \text{Spec}_1 \times \text{Spec}_2$$

Worked Example: Combining Tests, Boolean Method: MACE and SMC Likert Scale (3)

Sens and Spec for the combination of MACE and SMC Likert results [36] were calculated for the "AND" and "OR" combinations.

For the "AND" combination:

$$\text{Sens}_{\text{MACE"AND"SMC}} = \text{Sens}_{\text{MACE}} \times \text{Sens}_{\text{SMC}}$$
$$= 0.70 \times 0.90$$
$$= 0.63$$

$$\text{Spec}_{\text{MACE"AND"SMC}} = \text{Spec}_{\text{MACE}} + \left[(1 - \text{Spec}_{\text{MACE}}) \times \text{Spec}_{\text{SMC}} \right]$$
$$= 0.13 + [0.87 \times 0.36]$$
$$= 0.44$$

Looking at the 2×2 contingency table for series combination of MACE and SMC Likert (Fig. 8.3a), $\text{Sens}_{\text{MACE"AND"SMC}} = \text{TP}/(\text{TP} + \text{FN}) = 40/60 = 0.67$, and $\text{Spec}_{\text{MACE"AND"SMC}} = \text{TN}/(\text{FP} + \text{TN}) = 29/69 = 0.42$, both results similar to the above calculations.

For the "OR" combination:

$$\text{Sens}_{\text{MACE"OR"SMC}} = \text{Sens}_{\text{MACE}} + [(1 - \text{Sens}_{\text{MACE}}) \times \text{Sens}_{\text{SMC}}]$$
$$= 0.70 + [0.30 \times 0.90]$$
$$= 0.97$$

$$\text{Spec}_{\text{MACE"OR"SMC}} = \text{Spec}_{\text{MACE}} \times \text{Spec}_{\text{SMC}}$$
$$= 0.13 \times 0.36$$
$$= 0.05$$

Looking at the 2×2 contingency table for parallel combination of MACE and SMC Likert (Fig. 8.3b), $\text{Sens}_{\text{MACE"OR" SMC}} = \text{TP}/(\text{TP} + \text{FN}) = 54/60 = 0.93$, and $\text{Spec}_{\text{MACE"OR"SMC}} = \text{TN}/(\text{FP} + \text{TN}) = 5/69 = 0.07$, both results similar to the above calculations (Larner, unpublished observations).

Generally, sequential "AND" combination of tests leads to improvement in specificity, false positive rate, positive predictive value, and positive likelihood ratio. Conversely, sensitivity, false negative rate, negative predictive value and negative likelihood ratio are generally inferior with this method of combination ([38], p. 81–2, 133–6; [41], p. 119–43).

One possible advantage of the Boolean over the Bayesian method is that construction of a new 2 × 2 contingency table provides the opportunity to calculate many of the outcome measures discussed in previous chapters of this book for the combination of tests, not only post-test probability. For example, it is immediately evident (Fig. 8.4) that the combination of AD8 and 6CIT is sensitive for dementia diagnosis (0.82) with a high negative predictive value (0.90). The same technique has been used to combine the cognitive and executive functional subscores in Free-Cog, a hybrid screening instrument [46].

When more than two tests are involved, the Bayesian approach of multiplying the pre-test odds by the individual PLR values may become easier to apply than constructing new 2 × 2 contingency tables. However, this may conceal some shortcomings of combining tests.

Worked Example: Combining Tests, Bayesian Versus Boolean Methods: The Triple Test

The Attended With sign (AW), the Applause Sign (AS), and the Head-Turning Sign (HTS), have individually been noted as possible clinical markers of the presence of cognitive impairment. Their combination as the "Triple Test" to detect cognitive impairment has been suggested [26] and this has been examined in an independent dataset [39].

Of 85 patients administered all three tests, 44 were diagnosed with cognitive impairment based on clinical diagnostic criteria, hence pre-test probability (prevalence) of cognitive impairment in this cohort was 0.52, and pre-test odds (Sect. 1.3.3) was 1.07.

PLR for each sign was as follows (unpublished observations from data in [39]): $PLR_{AW} = 2.07$; $PLR_{AS} = 2.08$; and $PLR_{HTS} = 11.33$.

The results of the three tests were combined:

$$Post - test\ odds = Pre - test\ odds \times PLR_{AW} \times PLR_{AS} \times PLR_{HTS}$$
$$= 1.07 \times 2.07 \times 2.08 \times 11.33$$
$$= 52.19$$

This can be converted back to a post-test-probability using the equation:

$$Post - test\ probability = Post - test\ odds/(1 + post - test\ odds)$$
$$= 52.20/(1 + 52.20)$$
$$= 0.998$$

This combination of tests, the Triple Test, therefore shows a positive predictive value of 1, a marked improvement compared to the pre-test probability (0.52).

However, it may not be immediately evident from this Bayesian approach, but clear from the 2 × 2 contingency table constructed for the Boolean method (Fig. 8.5), that although both the PPV and specificity are perfect, the NPV is poor (0.5) and the sensitivity is negligible (0.07), with many false negatives, a pattern to be expected with the sequential "AND" combination of tests (Larner, unpublished observations). Many clinicians would find such test sensitivity unfit for purpose. The truth table for three tests combined using the "and" connective (Fig. 8.1a) also indicates the likelihood of many false negatives since so many of the outcomes are classified as negative.

		Diagnosis	
		Cognitive impairment present	Cognitive impairment absent
AW, AS, "AND" HTS outcome	All tests positive	True positive [TP] = 3	False positive [FP] = 0
	Any one negative	False negative [FN] = 41	True negative [TN] = 41

Fig. 8.5 2 × 2 contingency table for Triple Test (series combination of AW "AND" AS "AND" HTS) (N = 85) for the diagnosis of cognitive impairment (data from [39]). See also Fig. 8.1a

8.2.3   Decision Trees: "if-and-then" Rules

As these examples have shown, clinical problems may often be defined as staged processes consisting of successive dichotomous actions, concordant with the mode of clinical practice. Sequential testing strategies may be conveniently structured in the form of a decision tree.

Decision trees represent the chronological order of events with probabilities assigned to outcomes denoted by chance nodes (circles), to model uncertain events, and decision nodes (squares). Decision trees should incorporate all possible options (e.g. actions which may be chosen, or outcomes which may occur with each option) and hence extend beyond binary classification. Decision trees may be useful for the development of both diagnostic and prognostic predictions in the form of decision rules and algorithms. Such algorithms may permit standardization of approach but may also risk stifling innovation.

A clinical example is the cognitive disorders examination or Codex, a two-step decision tree for diagnostic prediction which incorporates results of two sequential tests (three-word recall and spatial orientation followed by a simplified clock drawing test) resulting in four terminal nodes with different probabilities of dementia diagnosis [6, 58]. Other, existing, screening instruments may be reformulated as decision trees (Mini-Cog [42]; Free-Cog [46]).

The dataset of the MACE and SMC Likert Scale study [36] (Sects. 8.2.1 and 8.2.2; Fig. 8.3a) may be reformatted as a simple decision tree (Fig. 8.6). Following the root node of "suspected cognitive impairment", the administration of tests is denoted by chance nodes (circles), modelling uncertain outcomes, with the continuous input variables collapsed into two categories according to test cut-off. Classifier diagnosis is denoted by decision nodes (squares), in this instance forming the terminal or leaf nodes of the tree. Decision trees may be arranged running from left to right, or from top to bottom, with the latter preferred here so that the terminal nodes may be seen to correspond to the rows of the 2×2 contingency table, both denoting classifier diagnosis (compare with Fig. 8.3a).

Decision trees may incorporate either absolute numbers or probabilities (see Fig. 8.6a, b respectively for the MACE "AND" SMC Likert Scale). That the order of tests gives the same classification is evident (Fig. 8.6c, an inversion of Fig. 8.6a), and the "OR" combination can also be represented (Fig. 8.6d; compare with Fig. 8.3b).

Although not part of typical decision trees, more distal "branches" or "leaves" have been added to these figures to show criterion diagnoses for comparison with the classifier diagnoses, information which permits summation of TP, FP, FN, and TN, and hence construction of "AND" and "OR" 2×2 contingency tables (Fig. 8.3).

Each path or route through the decision tree represents a classification decision rule, characterised by conditional statements: if condition 1 and condition 2 occur, then a specified outcome occurs. For example, in Fig. 8.6, if MACE $\leq 25/30$ and SMC $= 1-2$, then classifier diagnosis is cognitive impairment; but if MACE $\leq 25/30$ and SMC $= 3-5$ then, according to one classification rule, classifier diagnosis is no cognitive impairment (Fig. 8.6a), whereas following a different classification rule, classifier diagnosis is cognitive impairment (Fig. 8.6d). In these latter two particular instances, the two rules happen to be equivalent to the "AND" and "OR" Boolean classifiers.

The conditional statements underpinning a decision rule may also be conceptualised as an example of "if-and-then" patterns, rules, or algorithms. It has been suggested that such algorithms instantiate the neural mechanisms of discovery and invention [5]. A sequential classification decision rule, "if-and-and-and … then," accommodating as many "and" variables as required, will increase specificity, since it has more specifiers (as noted for sequential "AND" combination of tests; both are examples of causal operations). In the limiting iff case, "if-and-only-if–then," there is a single absolute specifier and hence specificity is perfect.

a) "AND" absolute numbers

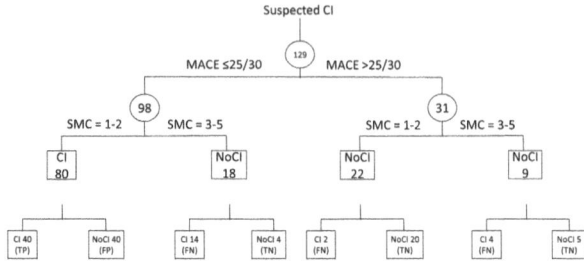

b) "AND" probabilities

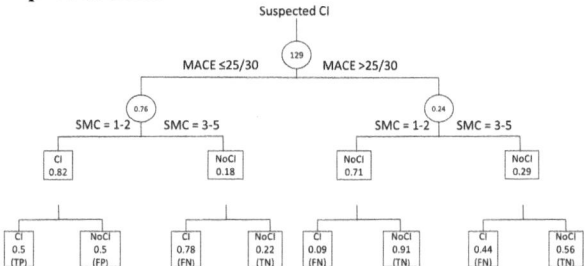

c) "AND" tree inverted

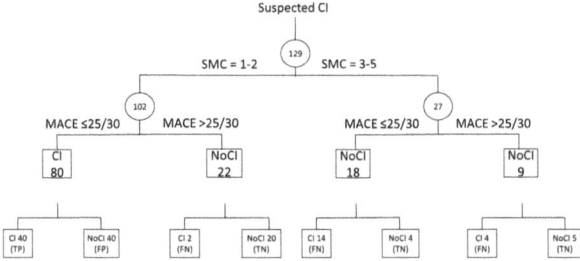

d) "OR" absolute numbers

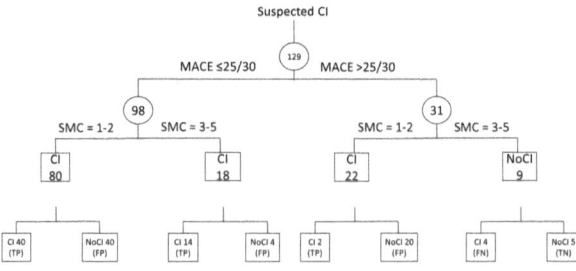

Fig. 8.6 Decision trees for combination of Mini-Addenbrooke's Cognitive Examination (MACE) and SMC Likert Scale outcomes (N = 129) for the diagnosis of cognitive impairment (data from [36]): a) "AND" absolute numbers; b) "AND" probabilities; c) "AND" tree inverted; d) "OR" absolute numbers

8.3   Effect Sizes

Measures of effect size, of which there are many, may be broadly categorised into measures of association (the r family), of which the phi (φ) coefficient (as Matthews' correlation coefficient) has already been described (Sect. 4.5), and differences between groups (the d family) [20]. The latter group, specifically Cohen's d, is the focus of this section.

8.3.1   Correlation Coefficient

Correlation coefficients, of which the best known is Pearson's product moment correlation coefficient (r), quantify the strength of relationship between two variables which may be either dichotomous or continuous. Correlations vary between $+1$ (perfect positive linear relationship) through 0 (no relationship between variables) to -1 (perfect negative linear relationship). It is well-recognised that correlation does not necessarily imply causation.

8.3.2   Cohen's d

Cohen's d effect size [13] is calculated as the difference of the means of the two groups being compared divided by the weighted pooled standard deviations of the groups (Fig. 8.7) if they are roughly the same (if not, then other options such as Glass's Δ or Hedges' g may be more appropriate [20]). Rules of thumb for the qualitative classification of Cohen's d effect size were given by Cohen [13, 14] and updated by Sawilowsky [53] (Table 8.1).

Hence Cohen's d is not calculated on the basis of the 2×2 contingency table; it is independent of cut point, and of base rate. Nevertheless, like AUC ROC (Sect. 7.2.2),

---

Cohen's d formula:

$$d = \frac{\overline{X}_1 - \overline{X}_2}{\sqrt{\dfrac{s_1^2 + s_2^2}{2}}}$$

Where d = Cohen's d effect size
X_1 and X_2 = means of two groups
s_1 and s_2 = standard deviations of two groups

Fig. 8.7 Cohen's d formula

Table 8.1 Classification of Cohen's d (after [13, 14, 53])

	Huge	Very large	Large	Medium	Small	Very poor
Cohen's d	≥2.00	≥1.20	≥0.80	≥0.50	≥0.20	≥0.01

Cohen's d quantifies the amount of separation between the distribution of scores for groups with and without the criterion diagnosis ([57], p. 208). Cohen's d may be used to compare between tests, such as cognitive screening instruments [31, 33], and values may change with disease prevalence [56].

Worked Examples: Cohen's d

In a large (N = 755) screening test accuracy study of MACE [37], a reference (criterion) diagnosis of dementia, based on the application of widely accepted diagnostic criteria for dementia, was made in 114 patients; the remaining patients without dementia (n = 641) had either mild cognitive impairment (MCI; n = 222) or subjective memory complaints (SMC; n = 419).

In the dementia group, mean MACE test score +/− standard deviation was 13.56 +/− 5.19. In the non-demented group, the mean score was 22.39 +/− 4.98. Hence;

$$d = 22.39 - 13.56/\sqrt{(5.19^2 + 4.98^2/2)}$$
$$= 8.83/5.09$$
$$= 1.74$$

According to the suggested classification of Cohen's d values (Table 8.1), this was a very large effect size.

Comparing MACE scores in the MCI group (mean = 19.09 +/− 4.78) with the SMC group (24.14 +/− 4.12):

$$d = 24.14 - 19.09/\sqrt{(4.78^2 + 4.12^2/2)}$$
$$= 5.05/4.46$$
$$= 1.13$$

According to the classification (Table 8.1), this was a large effect size [37].

To examine the change in various measures with disease prevalence, values were calculated for those aged ≥65 (n = 287) and ≥75 years (n = 119) comparing the dementia group with the non-dementia group [43]. In the ≥ 65 years group the mean MACE score in the dementia group was = 13.65 +/− 4.93 and in the non-dementia group it was 21.81 +/− 4.77. Hence calculating for Cohen's d:

$$d = 21.81 - 13.65/\sqrt{(4.93^2 + 4.77^2/2)}$$
$$= 8.16/4.85$$
$$= 1.68$$

According to the classification (Table 8.1), this was a very large effect size. For the ≥ 75 years group, mean MACE score in the dementia group was = 13.07 +/− 4.62 and in the non-dementia group was 19.58 +/− 4.37:

$$d = 19.58 - 13.07/\sqrt{(4.62^2 + 4.37^2/2)}$$
$$= 6.51/4.50$$
$$= 1.45$$

According to the classification (Table 8.1), this was a very large effect size (Larner, unpublished observations).

As both Cohen's d and r are standardised, they can be interconverted [20], e.g.

$$r = d/\sqrt{d^2 + 4}$$

8.3.3 Binomial Effect Size Display (BESD)

The binomial effect size display (BESD) is a 2×2 contingency table designed to present correlational effects in a manner indicating the "real-world" importance of the findings [51].

Correlation is expressed as a success rate difference, in rows expressing independent variables (e.g. treatment and control groups) and columns expressing any dependent variable which can be dichotomised (e.g. success, failure). For a given correlation, r, success rate is calculated for treatment and control groups as 0.5 +/− $r/2$, each column and row summing to 100. However, it has been argued that success rate differences may be biased by various factors and overestimate these values [25, 50].

Worked Example: Binomial Effect Size Display (BESD)

In the screening test accuracy study of MACE [37], it was found that for the diagnosis of dementia Cohen's d effect size = 1.74 (Sect. 8.3.2). To display this finding in a "real-world" manner, a binomial effect size display (BESD) was constructed. Firstly, r was calculated from Cohen's d:

$$r = d/\sqrt{d^2 + 4}$$
$$= 1.74/\sqrt{1.74^2 + 4}$$
$$= 0.656$$

For this correlation, success rate was calculated for patients diagnosed with and without dementia as $0.5 +/- r/2 = 0.172$ and 0.828. Hence, the BESD:

	Criterion diagnosis: dementia	Criterion diagnosis: no dementia
MACEdiagnosis: dementia	82.8	17.2
MACE diagnosis: no dementia	17.2	82.8

Diagnosis was therefore about five times more successful than unsuccessful. This gives a more optimistic result than the likelihood to be diagnosed or misdiagnosed (LDM) measure (Sect. 5.6): even at the optimal MACE cut-off defined by maximal LDM = NNM/NND, $\leq 15/30$ (Table 7.2), the unrounded LDM was only 3.94.

8.4 Other Measures of Association, Agreement, and Difference

8.4.1 McNemar's Test

The test first described by McNemar [47] examines paired nominal data in a 2×2 contingency table to determine whether row and column marginal frequencies are equal. It tests the null hypothesis of marginal homogeneity and hence is a measure of association.

In algebraic notation (see Fig. 1.2):

$$\chi^2 = (b - c)^2/(b + c)$$

This may sometimes be expressed by representing the larger number of pairs as n_1 and the smaller as n_2:

$$\chi^2 = (n_1 - n_2)^2/(n_1 + n_2)$$

When numbers are small ($b + c < 25$), a continuity correction is applied [19]:

$$\chi^2 = [(b - c) - 1]^2/(b + c)$$

or:

$$\chi^2 = [(n_1 - n_2) - 1]^2/(n_1 + n_2)$$

Worked Examples: McNemar Test of Association

In a study examining memory complaints in patients attending a dedicated epilepsy clinic ($N = 100$) [2], easily dichotomised screeners for both mood [4] and sleep disturbance [27, 28] were administered. There was a statistically significant difference in sleep disturbance and mood disturbance between the patients who reported subjective memory complaints and those who did not.

McNemar's test of association was used to examine whether there was a statistically significant association between disturbed sleep and disturbed mood in this patient cohort. Twenty patients had disturbed mood but not disturbed sleep ($= b$), whereas 6 patients had disturbed sleep but not disturbed mood ($= c$). Hence:

$$\chi^2 = (b - c)^2/(b + c)$$
$$= (20 - 6)^2/(20 + 6)$$
$$= 196/26$$
$$= 7.538$$
$$p = 0.009$$

Hence a statistically significant association between disturbed sleep and disturbed mood was found in this cohort of epilepsy patients, permitting rejection of the null hypothesis [2].

McNemar's test of association was used similarly in a study of patients diagnosed with functional cognitive disorders ($N = 44$) [7] to examine whether there was a statistically significant association between disturbed sleep and disturbed mood, using the same screeners for these constructs [4, 27, 28]. Five patients had disturbed mood but not disturbed sleep ($= b$), whereas 6 patients had disturbed sleep but not disturbed mood ($= c$). Hence, since $b + c < 25$, a continuity correction [19] was applied:

$$\chi^2 = [(b - c) - 1]^2/(b + c)$$

or, since $c > b$:

$$\chi^2 = [(n_1 - n_2) - 1]^2/(n_1 + n_2)$$

Let $n_1 = 6, n_2 = 5$:

$$\chi^2 = [(6-5)-1]^2/(6+5)$$
$$= 0/11$$
$$= 0$$
$$p = 1$$

Hence no statistically significant association between disturbed sleep and disturbed mood was found in this patient cohort [40].

Using data from the same study [7], the association between mood [4] and subjective memory complaint assessed with a dichotomised Likert scale [49] was also examined (N = 44). Four patients had disturbed mood but not subjective memory complaint (= b), whereas 8 patients had subjective memory complaint but not disturbed mood (= c). Again, a continuity correction was applied, since b + c < 25. As c > b, let $n_1 = 8, n_2 = 4$:

$$\chi^2 = [(n_1 - n_2) - 1]^2/(n_1 + n_2)$$
$$= [(8-4)-1]^2/(8+4)$$
$$= 9/12$$
$$= 0.75$$
$$p = 0.39$$

Hence no statistically significant association between subjective memory complaint and disturbed mood was found in this patient cohort [40].

Worked Example: McNemar Test of Association

Two brief cognitive screening instruments, the Mini-Cog [9] and the cognitive disorders examination (Codex) [6], were examined in a screening test accuracy study (N = 162) [42]. Using test cut-offs for dementia from the index studies, 16 patients categorised as "not dementia" by Codex were categorized as "dementia" by Mini-Cog (= b), whereas in only 3 patients was the reverse discordance observed (= c). Hence, since b + c <25, a continuity correction [19] was applied:

$$\chi^2 = [(b-c)-1]^2/(b+c)$$
$$= [(16-3)-1]^2/(16+3)$$
$$= 144/19$$

$$= 7.579$$

$$p = 0.0059$$

Hence the null hypothesis of marginal homogeneity was rejected. The marginal proportions were significantly different from each other. This is probably related to the better specificity of Codex than Mini-Cog for dementia diagnosis (Larner, unpublished observations).

As will be noted, McNemar's test is a test of the null hypothesis, with resultant conditional probability p values. The shortcomings of p values are well-recognised (Sect. 1.5), as they confound effect size with sample size, and a value "dichotomised" as significant at $p < 0.05$ is not a guarantee that a result is real (it could still be a false positive result or type I error), nor that a value deemed non-significant at $p > 0.05$ is inconclusive (it could still be a false negative result or type II error). The practice of using p values remains controversial, with some advocating their "retirement" [3].

8.4.2 Cohen's Kappa (κ) Statistic

The kappa statistic, κ, is usually designated as a measure of agreement or concordance beyond chance, for example between different observers, assessors or raters, or between different screening or diagnostic tests [15]. It may thus be conceptualised as a measure of precision rather than accuracy (but not precision understood as PPV; see Sects. 2.3.1 and 7.4.2). It is calculated by comparing the proportion of observed agreement, P_a, with the proportion of agreement expected by chance alone, P_c, for a total of N observations, where:

$$\kappa = (P_a - P_c)/(1 - P_c)$$

In algebraic notation (see Fig. 1.2):

$$P_a = (a + d)/N$$

Note that this corresponds to the definition previously given for Accuracy (Acc; Sect. 3.2.5). Hence this may also be expressed as:

$$\kappa = (Acc - P_c)/(1 - P_c)$$

The proportion of agreement expected by chance alone, P_c, is given by:

$$P_c = (a + b)(a + c)/N^2 + (c + d)(b + d)/N^2$$

Hence:

$$\kappa = (a + d)/N - \left[(a + b)(a + c)/N^2 + (c + d)(b + d)/N^2\right]$$
$$/1 - (a + b)(a + c)/N^2 + (c + d)(b + d)/N^2$$

or:

$$\kappa = 2(ad - bc)/[(a + c)(c + d) + (a + b)(b + d)]$$

κ ranges from $+1$ to -1, with most values expected to fall within the range 0 (agreement due to chance alone) to 1 (perfect agreement), with negative values occurring only when agreement occurs less often than predicted by chance alone, a rare situation in clinical practice. Interpretation of κ values is often based on the convention of Landis and Koch [29]: very good agreement (>0.8–1.0), good agreement (>0.6–0.8), moderate agreement (>0.4–0.6), fair agreement (>0.2–0.4), slight agreement (0–0.2), and poor agreement worse than chance (<0).

Worked Example: Accuracy with Kappa Statistic

In the screening test accuracy study of MACE [37], at the MACE cut-off of $\leq$20/30 the test outcomes were as follows: a (=TP) = 104, b (= FP) = 188, c (= FN) = 10, and d (= TN) = 453 (Fig. 2.2). Hence:

$$P_a = (a + d)/N$$
$$= 557/755$$
$$= 0.738$$
$$= \text{Acc (see Sect. 3.2.5)}$$

$$P_c = (a + b)(a + c)/N^2 + (c + d)(b + d)/N^2$$
$$= 292 \times 114/755^2 + 463 \times 641/755^2$$
$$= 33288/570025 + 296783/570025$$
$$= 0.0584 + 0.521$$
$$= 0.579$$

$$\kappa = (P_a - P_c)/(1 - P_c)$$
$$= (0.738 - 0.579)/(1 - 0.579)$$
$$= 0.159/0.421$$
$$= 0.378$$

Note that this result agrees with the calculation of unbiased Accuracy (UAcc = 0.378) shown in Sect. 3.2.7.

This may also be calculated using:

$$\kappa = 2(ad - bc)/[(a + c)(c + d) + (a + b)(b + d)]$$
$$= 2 \times 45232/[(114 \times 463) + (292 \times 641)]$$
$$= 2 \times 45232/52782 + 187172$$
$$= 90464/239954$$
$$= 0.377$$

[The different results relate to rounding errors.]

De Vet et al. [18] argued that Cohen's kappa is a relative measure, adjusting observed agreement for expected agreement, and hence is in fact a measure of reliability rather than a measure of agreement, hence accounting for the observation of instances of high agreement with low kappa and vice versa, for example in cases of class imbalance. Bangdiwala's B statistic is another summary measure of concordance.

Despite these caveats, Cohen's kappa may also be used for the comparison of assessors and the comparison of tests, as demonstrated in the following examples.

Worked Example: Cohen's Kappa (κ) Statistic – Comparison of Assessors

The Ascertain Dementia 8 (AD8) cognitive screening questionnaire was used in a study examining the frequency of cognitive impairment in patients with epilepsy [1]. AD8 may be administered to both patients [23] and informants [22]. The AD8 cut-off from the index studies was used, where a score $\geq 2/8$ indicates cognitive impairment is likely to be present.

In the study population (N = 100), there were 44 patient: informant dyads for whom both self-rated and informant AD8 scores were available. 21/44 patients self-rated AD8 $\geq 2/8$, and 24/44 informants rated patients' AD8 score $\geq 2/8$, with agreement in 21 dyads. 23/44 patients self-rated AD8 $<2/8$ and 20/44 informants rated patients' AD8 score $<2/8$, with agreement in 20 dyads. Constructing a 2×2 table the values for a, b, c, and d were therefore 21, 3, 0, and 20 respectively,

Hence observed agreement was:

$$P_a = (a + d)/N$$
$$= (21 + 20)/44$$
$$= 0.932$$

Agreement expected by chance was:

$$P_c = (a+b)(a+c)/N^2 + (c+d)(b+d)/N^2$$
$$= (21+3)(21+0)/44^2 + (0+20)(3+20)/44^2$$
$$= 0.260 + 0.238$$
$$= 0.498$$

Therefore:

$$\kappa = (P_a - P_c)/(1 - P_c)$$
$$= (0.932 - 0.498)/(1 - 0.498)$$
$$= 0.864$$

Based on the convention of Landis and Koch [29], this value of κ would be interpreted as very good agreement (>0.8–1.0).

Worked Example: Cohen's Kappa (κ) Statistic – Comparison of Screening Tests

Two cognitive screening instruments, the Mini-Addenbrooke's Cognitive Examination (MACE) [24] and the Montreal Cognitive Assessment (MoCA) [48], were examined in counterbalanced fashion in a screening test accuracy study [35] using cut-offs from the index studies of the tests (MACE ≤25/30; MoCA <26/30).

In the study population (N = 260), 182 had MACE scores ≤25/30 and 192 had MoCA scores <26/30. Constructing a 2 × 2 table, the values for a, b, c, and d were 164, 28, 18, and 50 respectively.

Hence observed agreement was:

$$P_a = (a+d)/N$$
$$= (164+50)/260$$
$$= 0.823$$

Agreement expected by chance was:

$$P_c = (a+b)(a+c)/N^2 + (c+d)(b+d)/N^2$$
$$= (164+28)(164+18)/260^2 + (18+50)(28+50)/260^2$$
$$= 0.517 + 0.078$$
$$= 0.595$$

Therefore:

$$\kappa = (P_a - P_c)/(1 - P_c)$$
$$= (0.823 - 0.595)/(1 - 0.595)$$
$$= 0.563$$

Based on the convention of Landis and Koch [29], this value of κ would be interpreted as moderate agreement (>0.4–0.6) (Larner, unpublished observations).

Kappa can be extended to encompass more than two categories and more than two raters, in which case some form of weighting may be required [16, 21].

In certain circumstances, kappa and Matthews' correlation coefficient (MCC; Sect. 4.5) coincide (symmetric matrix) [17], although these circumstances are unlikely to occur in clinical practice. Delgado and Tibau characterized kappa as the harmonic mean of the Youden index (Y; Sect. 4.2) and predictive summary index (PSI; Sect. 4.3) in this particular situation [17]; if so, this should be equivalent to the HMYPSI measure characterised previously (Sect. 4.4).

Worked Example: Kappa Statistic as Harmonic Mean of Y and PSI (HMYPSI)

In the screening test accuracy study of MACE [37], at the MACE cut-off of $\leq$20/30 the value of Y was 0.619 (Sect. 4.2) and of PSI was 0.334 (Sect. 4.3). If the kappa statistic is calculated as the harmonic mean of Y and PSI, then:

$$\kappa = 2/[1/Y + 1/PSI]$$
$$= 2.Y.PSI/(Y + PSI)$$
$$= 2 \times 0.619 \times 0.334/(0.619 + 0.334)$$
$$= 0.413/0.953$$
$$= 0.433$$
$$= HMYPSI \text{ (see Sect. 4.4)}$$

QED

Note that this result does not agree with the calculation of "Accuracy with kappa statistic" worked example (= 0.378), nor with the unbiased Accuracy (UAcc = 0.378) shown in Sect. 3.2.7. However, if the equation for kappa is re-written as:

$$\kappa = 2(ad - bc)/[(a + c)(b + d) + (a + b)(c + d)]$$

then using the data from the MACE study where a (=TP) = 104, b (=FP) = 188, c (=FN) = 10, and d (=TN) = 453, we obtain:

$$\kappa = 2(ad - bc)/[(a + c)(b + d) + (a + b)(c + d)]$$
$$= 2 \times 45232/[(114 \times 641) + (292 \times 463)]$$
$$= 2 \times 45232/73074 + 135196$$
$$= 90464/208270$$
$$= 0.434$$

[The different results relate to rounding errors.]

Hence the different result of "kappa statistic as harmonic mean of Y and PSI" compared to "Accuracy with kappa statistic" and "unbiased Acc" is a consequence of the different marginal totals. In the situation where b = c (i.e. a symmetric matrix) then the results would align, and would also be equal to the Matthews' correlation coefficient (Sect. 4.5).

Kappa statistic has shortcomings. It is affected by prevalence, and hence comparisons of its value determined in different populations may not be appropriate. As mentioned, it is also affected by class imbalance, when kappa scores may be low even when observed agreement is high. Moreover, kappa does not distinguish between types and sources of disagreement. It has been argued that the proportion of specific agreement, expressing the agreement separately for positive and negative ratings, is more clinically informative [18]. The first of these measures is identical to the F measure or Dice coefficient (Sect. 4.8.3). Some advocate that kappa should be avoided altogether [17]. Perhaps HMYPSI (Sect. 4.4) might be preferred, as it is an absolute measure rather than a relative measure.

8.4.3   Bland–Altman Method

Limits of agreement are not related to the 2 × 2 contingency table and are included here for completeness, in order to contrast with the previously described Cohen's kappa "measure of agreement". This is a method to provide a measure of agreement between tests by estimating how far apart the two values are on average and putting an interval around this [8]. The findings may be illustrated in a Bland–Altman plot of difference between test scores against their mean. The limits of agreement thus defined indicate how closely two methods agree, but what is accepted as "close" remains a clinical rather than a statistical judgement. The Bland–Altman methodology is a simple way to evaluate bias between mean differences which avoids the potentially erroneous conclusions based on correlation analyses [34].

8.5 Other Tables

8.5.1 Higher Order Tables

As previously discussed (Sect. 1.5), setting a decision threshold or dichotomisation point is critical to the construction of a 2×2 contingency table (potential methods for doing this are discussed in Sects. 7.3.1–7.3.6). This is not always a straightforward process. In clinical practice, dichotomisation may be inappropriate, for example when the object of tests is something other than simply identifying the presence or absence of disease. Furthermore, in screening or diagnostic test accuracy studies patients may not be tested with either the diagnostic test or the reference standard, or values may be lost or indeterminate. To accommodate the vagaries of real-world practice, it may be more appropriate to use larger contingency tables, such as 2×3 [54], 2×4 [12], or 3×3 ([52], p. 31), although this complicates the calculation of any of the measures previously discussed.

8.5.2 Interval Likelihood Ratios (ILRs)

An example of a higher order table may be provided by the use of interval likelihood ratios [11], as opposed to the more usual dichotomisation into positive and negative likelihood ratios (Sect. 2.3.5). Selecting the intervals is somewhat arbitrary, and the smaller the numbers in each interval the wider the confidence intervals (Sect. 1.7) are likely to be.

> **Worked Example: Higher Order Tables - Interval Likelihood Ratios**
>
> In the screening test accuracy study of MACE [37], category-specific positive and negative likelihood ratios were calculated at the MACE cut-off $\leq 20/30$, such that PLR = 3.11 and NLR = 0.124 at this cut-off (Sect. 2.3.5). However, looking at the spread of MACE scores in the whole patient study cohort (N = 755), as shown in Fig. 8.8, the overlap between dementia and no dementia patients extended over a range of MACE scores.

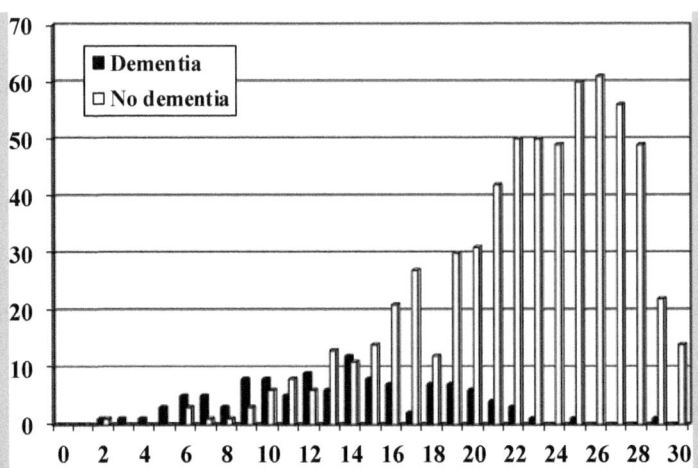

Fig. 8.8 MACE scores (x axis) by patient diagnosis (N = 755) (adapted from [37])

Although category-specific LRs may be calculated for each cut-off [37], another approach would be to calculate interval LRs (ILRs). For this purpose, a 2 × 5 table was constructed, from which ILRs were calculated, as TPR/FPR, or as $p(T+ \mid D +)/p(T+ \mid D-)$, as shown:

MACE score/30	Diagnosis: Dementia	Diagnosis: No dementia	Interval Likelihood Ratio (ILR)
26–30	1	202	(1/114)/(202/641) = 0.028
21–25	9	251	(9/114)/(251/641) = 0.202
16–20	29	121	(29/114)/(121/641) = 1.348
11–15	40	52	(40/114)/(52/641) = 4.325
≤10	35	15	(35/114)/(15/641) = 13.12
Total	**114**	**641**	

The ILR for MACE scores in the interval 26–30/30 was very small, 0.028, suggesting a very large change in probability (see Table 2.1 for a qualitative classification of LR values) and hence diagnostic gain for a diagnosis of no dementia. Likewise for the interval ≤10/30 the LR value, 13.12, was very large for a diagnosis of dementia. For the intervals 21–25/30 and 11–15/30 the LR values were qualitatively only moderate, although it should be noted that they represent an approximate change in probability of ±25% (Table 2.1 for a quantitative classification of LR values). The LR for the interval 16–20/30 was close to unity, suggesting only slight change in probability, and hence no diagnostic gain. This contrasts with the finding when the test was simply dichotomised at the cut-off ≤20/30. Results falling near a dichotomous cut-off may be distorted. The information from ILRs may assist clinical decision making to a greater extent than the simple dichotomised values for LR + and LR− (Larner, unpublished observations).

8.5.3 Three-Way Classification (Trichotomisation)

As previously mentioned (Sect. 1.6), three-way classification, or trichotomisation, is a method which may permit better classification accuracy by excluding or deselecting uncertain test scores, usually those falling near a dichotomous cut-off (Sect. 8.5.2), which are most error-prone. Unclassified individuals or instances may then require further assessment for correct classification. A downside of this approach is that calculation of sensitivity and specificity becomes cumbersome, being meant for dichotomous classification [30].

Worked Example: Three-Way Classification (Trichotomisation)

In the screening test accuracy study of MACE [37], result-specific likelihood ratios were calculated at all MACE cut-offs and plotted (Fig. 8.9).

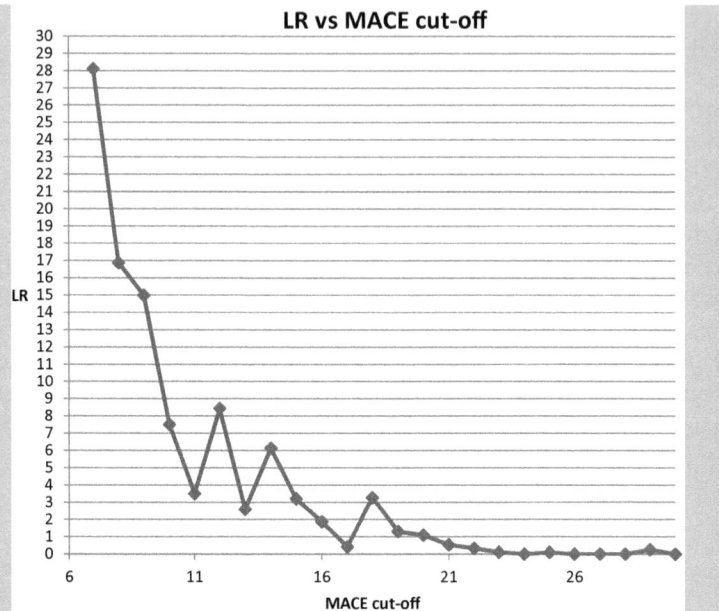

Fig. 8.9 Plot of result-specific likelihood ratios (LRs) on y axis versus MACE scores (x axis) for dementia diagnosis (data from [37]). Below MACE cut-off 6/30, LR values tend to ∞

If LR values >0.5 and <2 are considered to produce only a "slight" (decrease or increase respectively) in the probability of disease, whereas values ≤0.5 or ≥2 produce moderate change (Table 2.1), the former range might be deemed a zone of uncertainty. From the calculations and the plot it is possible to read off the range of MACE test scores corresponding to this range of LRs, namely ≤16/30 to ≤21/30 (the LR value at 18/30 is outside the 0.5 < LR < 2 range, but it is included here for convenience). This range contains 25.9% of all scores (196/755) and has an interval LR of (33/114)/(163/641) = 1.14. At the optimal MACE cut-off of ≤20/30, this range contains 63.1% of all the errors (4/10 false negatives, 121/188 false positives) (Larner, unpublished observations).

8.5.4 Fourfold Pattern of Risk Attitudes

Tversky and Kahneman noted that "the most distinctive implication of prospect theory is the fourfold pattern of risk attitudes" ([55], p. 306). Essentially this is a 2 × 2 contingency table cross-classifying gains and losses as classes against high and low probabilities as potential classifiers (Fig. 8.10). To preserve benefits, one may be risk averse for gains, whereas to avoid harms one may be risk seeking for losses.

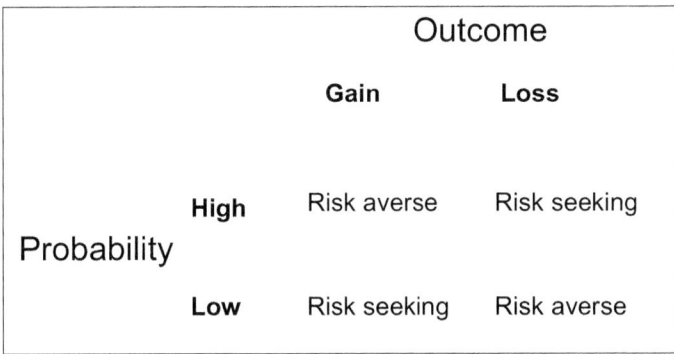

Fig. 8.10 The fourfold pattern of risk attitudes (after [53])

The fourfold pattern has applications in many fields, including economics and law, and is relevant to the net harm to net benefit (H/B) ratio (described in Sect. 2.3.6).

References

1. Aji BM, Larner AJ. Cognitive assessment in an epilepsy clinic using AD8 questionnaire. Epilepsy Behav. 2018;85:234–6.
2. Aji BM, Elhadd K, Larner AJ. Cognitive symptoms in people with epilepsy: role of sleep and mood disturbance. J Sleep Disord Ther. 2019;8:1.
3. Amrhein V, Greenland S, McShane B. Scientists rise up against statistical significance. Nature. 2019;567:305–7.
4. Arroll B, Khin N, Kerse N. Screening for depression in primary care with two verbally asked questions: cross sectional study. BMJ. 2003;327:1144–6.
5. Baron-Cohen S. The pattern seekers. A new theory of human invention. London: Penguin; 2022.
6. Belmin J, Pariel-Madjlessi S, Surun P, Bentot C, Feteanu D,Lefebvre des Noettes V, et al. The cognitive disorders examination (Codex) is a reliable 3-minute test for detection of dementia in the elderly (validation study in 323 subjects). Presse Med. 2007;36:1183–90.
7. Bharambe V, Larner AJ. Functional cognitive disorders: demographic and clinical features contribute to a positive diagnosis. Neurodegener Dis Manag. 2018;8:377–83.
8. Bland JM, Altman DG. Statistical methods for assessing agreement between two methods of clinical measurement. Lancet. 1986;1:307–10.
9. Borson S, Scanlan J, Brush M, Vitiliano P, Dokmak A. The Mini-Cog: a cognitive "vital signs" measure for dementia screening in multi-lingual elderly. Int J Geriatr Psychiatry. 2000;15:1021–7.
10. Brooke P, Bullock R. Validation of a 6 item cognitive impairment test with a view to primary care usage. Int J Geriatr Psychiatry. 1999;14:936–40.
11. Brown MD, Reeves MJ. Interval likelihood ratios: another advantage for the evidence-based diagnostician. Ann Emerg Med. 2003;42:292–7.
12. Burch J, Marson A, Beyer F, et al. Dilemmas in the interpretation of diagnostic accuracy studies on presurgical workup for epilepsy surgery. Epilepsia. 2012;53:1294–302.
13. Cohen J. Statistical power analysis for the behavioral sciences, 2nd ed. Hillsdale, New Jersey: Lawrence Erlbaum; 1988.

14. Cohen J. A power primer. Psychol Bull. 1992;112:155–9.
15. Cohen J. A coefficient of agreement for nominal scales. Educ Psychol Meas. 1960;20:37–46.
16. Cohen J. Weighted kappa: nominal scale agreement with provision for scaled disagreement or partial credit. Psychol Bull. 1968;70:213–20.
17. Delgado R, Tibau XA. Why Cohen's Kappa should be avoided as performance measure in classification. PLoS ONE. 2019;14(9): e0222916.
18. De Vet HCW, Mokkink LB, Terwee CB, Hoekstra OS, Knol DL. Clinicians are right not to like Cohen's κ. BMJ. 2013;346: f2515.
19. Edwards A. Note on the "correction for continuity" in testing the significance of the difference between correlated proportions. Psychometrika. 1948;13:185–7.
20. Ellis PD. The essential guide to effect sizes: statistical power, meta-analysis, and the interpretation of research results. Cambridge: Cambridge University Press; 2010.
21. Fleiss JL. Measuring nominal scale agreement among many raters. Psychol Bull. 1971;76:378–82.
22. Galvin JE, Roe CM, Xiong C, Morris JE. Validity and reliability of the AD8 informant interview in dementia. Neurology. 2006;67:1942–8.
23. Galvin JE, Roe CM, Coats MA, Morris JC. Patient's rating of cognitive ability: using the AD8, a brief informant interview, as a self-rating tool to detect dementia. Arch Neurol. 2007;64:725–30.
24. Hsieh S, McGrory S, Leslie F, Dawson K, Ahmed S, Butler CR, et al. The Mini-Addenbrooke's Cognitive Examination: a new assessment tool for dementia. Dement Geriatr Cogn Disord. 2015;39:1–11.
25. Hsu LM. Biases of success rate differences shown in binomial effect size displays. Psychol Methods. 2004;9:183–97.
26. Isik AT, Soysal P, Kaya D, Usarel C. Triple test, a diagnostic observation, can detect cognitive impairment in older adults. Psychogeriatrics. 2018;18:98–105.
27. Jenkins CD, Stanton BA, Niemcryk SJ, Rose RM. A scale for the estimation of sleep problems in clinical research. J Clin Epidemiol. 1988;41:313–21.
28. Lallukka T, Dregan A, Armstrong D. Comparison of a sleep item from the General Health Questionnaire-12 with the Jenkins Sleep Questionnaire as measures of sleep disturbance. J Epidemiol. 2011;21:474–80.
29. Landis JR, Koch GG. The measurement of observer agreement for categorical data. Biometrics. 1977;33:159–74.
30. Landsheer JA. Impact of prevalence of cognitive impairment on the accuracy of the Montreal Cognitive Assessment. The advantage of using two MoCA thresholds to identify error-prone test scores. Alzheimer Dis Assoc Disord. 2020;34:248–53.
31. Larner AJ. Effect size (Cohen's d) of cognitive screening instruments examined in pragmatic diagnostic accuracy studies. Dement Geriatr Cogn Disord Extra. 2014;4:236–41.
32. Larner AJ. AD8 informant questionnaire for cognitive impairment: pragmatic diagnostic test accuracy study. J Geriatr Psychiatry Neurol. 2015;28:198–202.
33. Larner AJ. Cognitive screening instruments for the diagnosis of mild cognitive impairment. Prog Neurol Psychiatry. 2016;20(2):21–6.
34. Larner AJ. Correlation or limits of agreement? Applying the Bland-Altman approach to the comparison of cognitive screening instruments. Dement Geriatr Cogn Disord. 2016;42:247–54.
35. Larner AJ. MACE versus MoCA: equivalence or superiority? Pragmatic diagnostic test accuracy study. Int Psychogeriatr. 2017;29:931–7.
36. Larner AJ. Dementia screening: a different proposal. Future Neurol. 2018;13:177–9.
37. Larner AJ. MACE for diagnosis of dementia and MCI: examining cut-offs and predictive values. Diagnostics (Basel). 2019;9:E51.
38. Larner AJ. Diagnostic test accuracy studies in dementia. A pragmatic approach. 2nd ed. London: Springer; 2019.
39. Larner AJ. Response to "Triple test, a diagnostic observation, can detect cognitive impairment in older adults." Psychogeriatrics. 2019;19:407–8.
40. Larner AJ. Functional cognitive disorders: update on diagnostic status. Neurodegener Dis Manag. 2020;10:67–72.

41. Larner AJ. Manual of screeners for dementia. Pragmatic test accuracy studies. London: Springer; 2020.
42. Larner AJ. Mini-Cog versus Codex (cognitive disorders examination): is there a difference? Dement Neuropsychol. 2020;14:128–33.
43. Larner AJ. Mini-Addenbrooke's Cognitive Examination (MACE): a useful cognitive screening instrument in older people? Can Geriatr J. 2020;23:199–204.
44. Larner AJ. Combining results of performance-based and informant test accuracy studies: Bayes or Boole? Dement Geriatr Cogn Disord. 2021;50:29–35.
45. Larner AJ. Wittgenstein, neurology and neuroscience. Brain. 2022;145:3–6.
46. Larner AJ, Burns A. Free-Cog reformulated: analyses as independent or stepwise tests of cognitive and executive function. medRxiv. https://doi.org/10.1101/2023.01.29.23285153.
47. McNemar Q. Note on the sampling error of the difference between correlated proportions or percentages. Psychometrika. 1947;12:153–7.
48. Nasreddine ZS, Phillips NA, Bédirian V, Charbonneau S, Whitehead V, Collin I, et al. The Montreal Cognitive Assessment, MoCA: a brief screening tool for mild cognitive impairment. J Am Geriatr Soc. 2005;53:695–9.
49. Paradise MB, Glozier NS, Naismith SL, Davenport TA, Hickie IB. Subjective memory complaints, vascular risk factors and psychological distress in the middle-aged: a cross-sectional study. BMC Psychiatry. 2011;11:108.
50. Randolph JJ, Edmondson RS. Using the binomial effect size display to present the magnitude of effect sizes to the evaluation audience. Pract Assess Res Eval. 2005;10:14.
51. Rosenthal R, Rubin DR. A simple, general purpose display of magnitude of experimental effect. J Educ Psychol. 1982;74:166–9.
52. Sackett DL, Haynes RB. The architecture of diagnostic research. In: Knottnerus JA, editor. The evidence base of clinical diagnosis. London: BMJ Books; 2002. p. 19–38.
53. Sawilowsky SS. New effect sizes rules of thumb. J Mod Appl Stat Methods. 2009;8:597–9.
54. Schuetz GM, Schlattmann F, Dewey M. Use of 3×2 tables with an intention to diagnose approach to assess clinical performance of diagnostic tests: meta-analytical evaluation of coronary CT angiography studies. BMJ. 2012;345: e6717.
55. Tversky A, Kahneman D. Advances in prospect theory: cumulative representation of uncertainty. J Risk Uncertain. 1992;5:297–323.
56. Wojtowicz A, Larner AJ. Diagnostic test accuracy of cognitive screeners in older people. Prog Neurol Psychiatry. 2017;21(1):17–21.
57. Youngstrom EA. A primer on receiver operating characteristic analysis and diagnostic efficiency statistics for pediatric psychology: we are ready to ROC. J Pediatr Psychol. 2014;39:204–21.
58. Ziso B, Larner AJ. Codex (cognitive disorders examination) decision tree modified for the detection of dementia and MCI. Diagnostics (Basel). 2019;9:E58.

Chapter 9
Classification of Metrics of Binary Classification

Contents

9.1   Introduction

The previous chapters in this book have described a wide range of measures used to describe the outcomes of contingency tables, mostly of the 2×2 confusion matrix variety but some of higher order. In this final chapter, possible ways to classify the various measures of binary classification are considered, as a prelude to investigate briefly the nature of uncertainty and the measures best used to address it.

9.2   Classification of Metrics of Binary Classification

The many measures discussed in previous chapters of this book may be classified in many different ways, which are not necessarily mutually exclusive. Clinician preferences for particular measures may be based on some, all, or none of these considerations, which may be conceptualised as metaclassifications.

9.2.1   Error/Information/Association-Based

The classification of measures suggested by Bossuyt [3] as error-based, information-based, or association-based was adopted in Chaps. 2, 3, and 6. Hence sensitivity, specificity, accuracy and their complements may be classified as error-based; predictive values, likelihood ratios, and predictive ratios may be classified as information-based; and diagnostic odds ratios and clinical utility indexes may be classified as association-based.

9.2.2   Descriptive Versus Predictive

Measures might also be distinguished as descriptive (e.g. sensitivity, specificity) or predictive (e.g. predictive values or ratios). As predictive power is a marker of science, the latter might seem preferable, but as noted these values are dependent on prevalence and hence may be difficult to generalise.

9.2.3   Statistical: Frequentist Versus Bayesian

A classification based on statistical considerations lies between frequentist and Bayesian approaches. Frequentist approaches assign probabilities to data whereas Bayesian approaches assign probabilities to hypotheses and incorporate prior knowledge, updating this as more data become available. Since diagnostic reasoning is (ideally) hypothesis driven, the Bayesian approach may seem more appropriate in clinical situations, and hence measures such as predictive values and likelihood ratios, post-test odds and net harm to net benefit ratio, may be preferred compared to sensitivity, specificity, and area under the receiver operating characteristic curve (AUC ROC).

9.2.4 Test-oriented Versus Patient-Oriented

Measures may also be classified as test-oriented or patient-oriented. The former grouping includes sensitivity and specificity (see Chap. 2) and the ROC curve (Chap. 7) but, as has been pointed out [7], these measures do not answer clinicians' questions, being orientated to the test rather than to the patient. The latter grouping includes predictive values (see Chap. 2) and "number needed" measures (Chap. 5). Examples of measures which attempt to combine test- and patient-oriented measures include clinical utility indexes (Chap. 2), HMYPSI, MCC, CSI, F, and SUI (Chap. 4).

9.2.5 Range

Another empirical classification may be suggested, according to the possible range of test scores.

From 0 to 1: this includes all conditional probabilities such as sensitivity, specificity, predictive values, accuracy and their complements (with which they sum to 1). These probabilities might be expressed as percentages, although there is evidence that this can lead to confusion for clinicians [2] and hence the use of values from 0 to 1 in this text.

These values are unscaled, and hence may be influenced by prevalence (predictive values), cut-off or level of the test (sensitivity and specificity), or both (accuracy), although attempts to scale these values may be made. The area under the ROC curve also falls within this group defined by test range.

From −1 to +1: Unitary or global measures which try to combine some of the paired measures discussed in the previous section may have a range from −1 to 1, e.g. the Youden index (Y), which combines sensitivity and specificity; the predictive summary index (PSI) which combines positive and negative predictive values; the identification index (II) which combines accuracy and inaccuracy; the Matthews' correlation coefficient (MCC) which encompasses sensitivity, specificity, and positive and negative predictive values.

The implications of the extended score range are that a value $= 0$ denotes a useless test, a value of $+1$ indicates a perfect classifier, whilst values <0 indicate disagreement between prediction and observation.

Some of these measures may be normalized to give a range from 0 to 1, e.g. Y as balanced accuracy (Sect. 3.2.6), MCC as normalized MCC (Sect. 4.5).

From 0 to 2: Few measures encompass this range, e.g. the sum of sensitivity and specificity, sometimes called the "gain in certainty," a measure seldom used. This is also known as the overall correct classification rate (Sect. 3.2.4). The misclassification rate, based on the complements of sensitivity and specificity, also has a range of 0 to 2 and is the complement of Y. The "summary utility index" (SUI), based on clinical utility indexes, also falls in this group.

***From 0 to infinity (but not beyond!)*:** Global measures which try to combine some of the paired measures in the form of odds ratios have a range from 0 to ∞, such as likelihood ratios, diagnostic odds ratios, and the various forms of the efficiency index. These have inflection points at 1.

***Others*:** outliers include the likelihood to diagnose or predict measures (Sects. 5.6 and 5.7), which because of the method of their construction have a range from -1 to ∞.

9.3 Conclusion

9.3.1 Fourfolds, Uncertainty, and the Epistemological Matrix

Many examples of the "rule of four" or the "law of four," such as Byrhtferth's diagram, may be found in cultural history (likewise rules or systems of three or of five) ([22], p. 210–4, 219, 236–7), likewise fourfold structures in the history of philosophy ([9], p. 79). However, "we need to be careful not to assume that all … quadruple structures are alike, since the only thing that fourfolds usually share in common is that they result from two separate principles of division. … the mere existence of a fourfold structure does not prove that anything interesting has been discovered – which would require that the two axes of division are both relevant to their subject *and* somewhat surprising in their conclusions" ([10], p. 150–1). In the process of developing Heidegger's *das Geviert*, Harman proposes two criteria to judge the success of laying two binary oppositions crosswise ([9], p. 80):

- How well chosen are the two axes of division?
- Does a given fourfold system provide a useful account of how the four poles interrelate?

It is possible, for example, to characterise the Hippocratic-Galenic humoural theory, which dominated medical thinking for around two millennia [1], as a 2 × 2 table, cross-classifying pairs of qualities (hot/cold, wet/dry) to derive the four humours and their associated temperaments (Fig. 9.1). Applying Harman's criteria from our (privileged) standpoint in medical history, we might take the view that however useful an account the humoural system might give, the axes are ill chosen since they give "little instruction as to how the [medical] universe works," as reflected in the lack of evidence for therapeutic efficacy using such a system.

"What do I know?" asked Montaigne (1533–1592) in his *Essais*. Do we know, or simply think we know? Is there an objective knowledge, which we may only perceive subjectively, as through a prism, through the medium of the workings of our brain? "We do not look at things as they are, but as we are" said Kant (1724–1804).

Such reflections might also be summarised in a 2 × 2 table, which I have ventured to call an epistemological matrix ([15], p. 157–8) (Fig. 9.2), and which may have relevance not only to that sphere of philosophy (as all knowledge is historically

Paired qualities		Hot	Cold
Paired qualities	Wet (moist, humid)	Blood, sanguine	Phlegm, phlegmatic
	Dry	Yellow bile, choleric	Black bile, melancholic

Fig. 9.1 Classical humoural theory reformulated as a 2 × 2 contingency table

contingent) but also to psychology. It takes uncertainty as inherent to the human condition, with marked class imbalance due to the predominance of the unknown column, and to the unknown unknown category in particular. We are blind to our blindness, and have an almost unlimited ability to ignore our ignorance ([11], p. 24, 201); "unobservables cannot be detected, and are epistemically unavailable" [23]. Consider, for example, the experiential and intellectual limitations of the residents of Edwin Abbott's two-dimensional *Flatland* (even the pentagonal-shaped doctors!). Here one might also include the anoetic or nonknowing consciousness proposed by Tulving, encompassing abilities such as implicit memory (we all have a degree of cognitive anosognosia). The omniscient lies outside the matrix.

		Objectivity	
		Known	Unknown
Subjectivity	Known	Known Known	Known Unknown
	Unknown	Unknown Known	Unknown Unknown

Fig. 9.2 The (2 × 2) epistemological matrix (revised from [15], p. 157)

		Understanding	
		Present	**Absent**
Conscious Awareness	**Present**	Certainty	Uncertainty
	Absent	Knowledge	Ignorance

Fig. 9.3 Relationship of epistemic states (adapted from [8], p. 15)

This suggested epistemological 2 $\times$ 2 matrix formulation may overlap with the relationship between uncertainty and other epistemic states as tabulated by Han [8] which cross-classifies understanding with conscious awareness (Fig. 9.3).

This approach may permit a reformulation of the original epistemological matrix, since certainty and uncertainty are considered as metacognitive subjective states of awareness (Fig. 9.4). The appeal to metacognition is significant not only philosophically but also clinically, as disordered metacognition may be pertinent to many clinical presentations, as in functional neurological disorders [16]. Moreover, this reformulation in terms of uncertainty emphasizes the fuzziness of boundaries (epistemic thresholds; Sect. 1.4) between the cells: rather than categorically distinct, either/or characteristics, these are qualities which vary along a continuum ([8], p. 100).

		Understanding		
		Present	**Absent**	
Conscious awareness	**Present**	Known known = Certainty	Known unknown = Uncertainty	Metacognitive (subjective) states
	Absent	Unknown known = Knowledge	Unknown unknown = Ignorance	Cognitive states

Fig. 9.4 The (2 $\times$ 2) epistemological matrix (Fig. 9.2) revised in light of Han's formulation of epistemic states (Fig. 9.3)

9.3.2   Which Measure(s) Should Be Used?

"As in any sorting-out process, Roget was plagued by the big problem inherent in classification: the validity of categories vs. the continuum of nature" ([5], p. 268).

As I have learned more over the years, I have been intrigued by the number of measures which may be derived from an ostensibly simple 2×2 grid and by their interrelationships. This presumably reflects, at least in part, the internally coherent, self-sustaining, nature of (elementary) mathematical methods. Unless inadvertently unaware of prior accounts, I have added several new measures to this number [14, 15], including: PCDI, NCDI (Sect. 2.4.3); Balanced Level values (Sect. 3.3.3); HMYPSI (Sect. 4.4); SUI, SDI (Sect. 4.9); LDM, LPM, NNCC, NNMC, LCM, EI and variants, NNSU, NNSD, LSUD, (Chap. 5); and various quality measures (Chap. 6).

The analysis offered in this book has been restricted, in the interests of simplicity and by the author's limited abilities, to binary classification. This is recognised to have shortcomings (e.g. loss of information, Sects. 1.5, 1.6, and 8.5.1; misclassi- fication, Sect. 3.2.4) and potential solutions (e.g. higher order tables, Sect. 8.5.1; trichotomisation, Sects. 1.6 and 8.5.3) although these may not be straightforward to apply. Moreover, correct construction of 2×2 tables and calculation of outputs does not obviate the necessity to assess risk of bias (internal validity) and generalis- ability of findings (external validity). However, in medical practice, dichotomisation is pragmatic for clinical decision making [7], and hence likely to continue, since "Probabilities can only guide the determination of whether a patient does or does not have a disease" ([6], p. 164). As previously stated (Sect. 1.7), these various measures allow us to substitute an approximate generalisation for an absolute rule, except in (the unusual) limit cases where the absolute rule holds (e.g. Sens = 1, PPV =1, Acc = 1, i.e. FNR = 0, FDR = 0, Inacc = 0; EI = ∞).

How, then, should one steer a course through the many summary measures which have been described in this text? What measure(s) should be selected for analysis of a study? This may depend in part on the particular question being asked, the context, and also familiarity, personal preference (what one finds most intuitive, or easily communicable to patients), and fashion. In clinical medicine the F measure and Matthews' correlation coefficient are seldom used [12, 13] whereas the former is almost obligatory in information retrieval and machine learning contexts, despite its recognised shortcomings [20].

The outputs of meta-analyses are usually given in terms of summary sensitivity and specificity and ROC curve but these measures do not answer clinicians' questions, being orientated to the test rather than to the patient [7]. Predictive values, being orientated to the patient, might seem more clinically useful but these values are unstable because of their dependence on prevalence. Positive and negative likelihood ratios may obviate these problems, but dichotomisation risks loss of information and distortion, and calculation of interval likelihood ratios is more involved and the choice of intervals may be arbitrary.

As stated in the Introductory chapter (Sect. 1.7), it might be intuited that the very multiplicity of the measures which may be derived from 2×2 contingency tables suggests their inadequacy, if summary statistics reduce the information to a single characteristic of the data. Is there a minimum set or a standard "dashboard" [21], a limited set of measures which shows what "really matters" (i.e. guides what we do) and hence which might be agreed by expert consensus? None yet exists, to my knowledge.

Both the STAndards for the Reporting of Diagnostic accuracy studies guideline (STARD [4]) and its iteration for studies in dementia (STARDdem [19]) recommended sensitivity and specificity as keywords of papers reporting diagnostic test accuracy studies. Likelihood ratios may be used as the basis for recommendations about suitable tests (e.g. for dementia [18]). Some measures may be preferred as test-oriented (Sens, Spec, FPR, FNR, LRs), or patient-oriented (PPV, NPV, predictive ratios), or as indices of validity (LR, DOR, Y), or as more intuitive (Net reclassification improvement, "Number needed to" measures). Test shortcomings, as evidenced by the use of error notation (Sect. 1.4) wherever appropriate throughout this book, may also be denoted by what I have ventured to term "metrics of limitation" [17] such as false rates (positive, negative, discovery, reassurance; Sects. 2.2.2 and 2.3.2), misclassification rate (Sect. 3.2.4), net harm to net benefit (H/B) ratio (Sect. 2.3.6), likelihood to be diagnosed or misdiagnosed (Sect. 5.6), and clinical disutility indexes (Sect. 2.4.3). Quality measures (Chap. 6) may reduce the risk of overoptimistic interpretation of results. Many of these various measures may be less familiar, and outside clinician literacy, but this could be addressed if the measures were deemed sufficiently useful, for example in communicating information to patients. Ultimately, the provision of test datasets should allow researchers to calculate any parameter of interest not explicitly stated in the index paper.

"Ars longa vita brevis" wrote Hippocrates (or one of his followers). The art of medicine may be, for the gifted, an intuitive process, but for others the art is long and deliberative. Intuitive thinking may be liable to error [11]. The use of the measures described in this book may assist deliberative medical decision making and the avoidance of error, and also find application in other disciplines as well.

References

1. Arikha N. Passions and tempers. A history of the humours. New York: Harper Perennial; 2008.
2. Bodemer N, Meder B, Gigerenzer G. Communicating relative risk changes with baseline risk: presentation format and numeracy matter. Med Decis Making. 2014;34:615–26.
3. Bossuyt PMM. Clinical validity: defining biomarker performance. Scand J Clin Lab Invest. 2010;70(Suppl242):46–52.
4. Bossuyt PM, Reitsma JB, Bruns DE, et al. The STARD statement for reporting studies of diagnostic accuracy: explanation and elaboration. Clin Chem. 2003;49:7–18.
5. Emblen DJ. Peter Mark Roget. The word and the man. London: Longman; 1970.
6. Freidson E. Profession of medicine. A study of the sociology of applied knowledge. New York: Dodd, Mead; [1970] 1975.
7. Gallagher EJ. The problem with sensitivity and specificity... Ann Emerg Med. 2003;42:298–303.

8. Han PKJ. Uncertainty in medicine. A framework for tolerance. Oxford: Oxford University Press; 2021.
9. Harman G. The quadruple object. Winchester: Zer0 Books; 2011.
10. Harman G. Object-oriented ontology. A new theory of everything. London: Pelican; 2018.
11. Kahneman D. Thinking, fast and slow. London: Penguin; 2012.
12. Larner AJ. What is test accuracy? Comparing unitary accuracy metrics for cognitive screening instruments. Neurodegener Dis Manag. 2019;9:277–81.
13. Larner AJ. Defining "optimal" test cut-off using global test metrics: evidence from a cognitive screening instrument. Neurodegener Dis Manag. 2020;10:223–30.
14. Larner AJ. Manual of screeners for dementia. Pragmatic test accuracy studies. London: Springer; 2020.
15. Larner AJ. The 2 × 2 matrix. Contingency, confusion and the metrics of binary classification. London: Springer; 2021.
16. Larner AJ. Functional cognitive disorders (FCD): how is metacognition involved? Brain Sci. 2021;11(8):1082.
17. Larner AJ. Cognitive screening instruments for dementia: comparing metrics of test limitation. Dement Neuropsychol. 2021;15:458–63.
18. National Institute for Health and Care Excellence. Dementia. Assessment, management and support for people living with dementia and their carers. NICE Guideline 97. Methods, evidence and recommendations (https://www.nice.org.uk/guidance/ng97). London: NICE; 2018.
19. Noel-Storr AH, McCleery JM, Richard E, et al. Reporting standards for studies of diagnostic test accuracy in dementia: the STARDdem initiative. Neurology. 2014;83:364–73.
20. Powers DMW. What the F measure doesn't measure … Features, flaws, fallacies and fixes. 2015; 1503.06410.2015.
21. Stiglitz JE. Measuring what matters. Sci Am. 2020;323(2):20–7.
22. Strevens M. The knowledge machine. How an unreasonable idea created modern science. London: Penguin; 2020.
23. Thiebaut de Schotten M, Foulon C, Nachev P. Brain disconnections link structural connectivity with function and behaviour. Nat Commun. 2020;11:5094.

Index